Fetal Growth in Humans

Herbert C. Miller, M.D.
Professor of Pediatrics
University of Kansas Medical
 Center, College of Health
 Sciences and Hospital
Kansas City, Kansas

T. Allen Merritt, M.D.
Assistant Professor of Pediatrics
 and of Obstetrics and Gynecology
University of Rochester School of
 Medicine and Dentistry
Rochester, New York

YEAR BOOK MEDICAL PUBLISHERS, INC.
CHICAGO • LONDON

Library of Congress Cataloging in Publication Data

Miller, Herbert C
    Fetal growth in humans.

    Includes index.
    1. Fetus — Growth. 2. Fetus — Growth retardation.
I. Merritt, T. Allen, joint author. II. Title.
[DNLM: 1. Infant, Newborn. 2. Fetal growth
retardation — Etiology. WQ211 M648f]
RG600.M54   618.3'2   79-9974
ISBN 0-8151-5907-2

Acknowledgments

THE FETAL GROWTH RESEARCH PROGRAM that provided most of the data used in this text was undertaken with the full cooperation of Kermit Krantz, M.D., Chairman and Professor in the Department of Gynecology and Obstetrics, The University of Kansas Medical Center, College of Health Sciences and Hospital, and the members of his department. Approval for the research program was given by the Human Ethics Committee of The University of Kansas Medical Center. We gratefully acknowledge the assistance of Thomas Clarke, M.D., Fellow in Perinatology, University of California, San Diego, in the preparation of parts of this manuscript. Grace Holmes, M.D., Assistant Professor of Pediatrics, The University of Kansas Medical Center, College of Health Sciences and Hospital, was responsible for the long-term follow-up studies carried out in conjunction with the Fetal Growth Research Program, on which most of this text was based. The data presented here on the postnatal growth of undergrown fetuses are the result of her studies. Without her participation, this portion of the study could not have been done. Khatab Hassanein, Ph.D., Chairman and Professor in the Department of Biometry, The University of Kansas Medical Center, College of Health Sciences and Hospital, has from the beginning contributed heavily to the statistical evaluation of data collected in the Fetal Growth Research Program. We thank him for his valuable help with the statistics in this text. The senior author is particularly indebted to his secretary, Susan LeClaire, who cheerfully and expeditiously constructed innumerable tables and typed the several revisions of the text. He is also grateful for the generous support provided him by the Mead Johnson Co. of Evansville, Indiana, over the period of 5 years covered by the study of fetal growth at The University of Kansas Medical Center.

Contents

Introduction

A STUDY OF FETAL GROWTH in all infants born at The University of Kansas Medical Center was begun by the senior author in March, 1973. The study involved taking body measurements of all infants at birth (almost always within the first 48 hours after birth) by him and correlating these measurements with a large number of factors in the mothers' medical and obstetric records and with the infants' hospital records. All mothers were interviewed before discharge from the hospital to learn about their smoking habits during pregnancy and to check on any part of their medical and obstetric records that might be unclear, unstated or questionable. Information that mothers gave about their smoking habits correlated well with the number of cigarette butts in their bedside ashtrays. Approximately 6000 black and white mothers and their infants were thus observed over a period of the next 5 years. In about 10% of those observed, the information was not completed for one reason or another, usually because the mothers were referred in from some distance away from the Medical Center and their prenatal data were delayed in arrival or incomplete. Vacations and indispositions of the senior author interrupted the collection of data from time to time. Data on large numbers of mothers involved with a specific area of interest were computerized. Data relating to special areas of interest involving small numbers of mothers were not computerized.

It is believed that the 5 years covered by the study provided a population of mothers and infants that is unique in the annals of fetal growth in humans in that the measurements and evaluations of the newborn infants and the collection of data on the mothers were done by one person. The population included mothers who experienced a wide range of socioeconomic circumstances, of medical and obstetric problems and of behavioral attitudes relating to their pregnancies. The population cannot be said to be representative of populations at large. The mothers were mostly from a large urban setting of more than 1,000,000 people. But this is a tertiary medical center and, as might be expected, the incidence of mothers with special medical and social problems undoubtedly was high as compared to the population at large. We do not see that the skewness of the population of mothers admitted to this Medical Center for delivery has been a handicap, because we have grouped mothers according to their medical, obstetric and social backgrounds, and have tried to take advantage of their skewness.

There was need for a large population of mothers and infants in order to have enough mothers with only a single known growth-retarding factor in their pregnancies, which would permit for the first time a study to be made of the effects of a single factor. Previous literature has dealt with single growth-retarding factors, but it is apparent in presenting their effects on fetal growth and pregnancy outcome that not all known growth-retarding factors had been taken into account and removed. In clinical practice, obstetricians are confronted frequently with a number of fetal growth-retarding variables in a single pregnancy. Obstetricians need to know what the effects are on the fetus not only of a single but also of multiple growth-retarding factors. Our study makes clear that the risk to the fetus depends on the number of fetal growth-retarding factors present in the mother's pregnancy. Despite a comparatively large number of mothers in the study, we were able to find but a few women who were chronic alcoholics or involved with addicting drugs or totally lacking in prenatal care. Large numbers of mothers were also needed to find enough women whose pregnancies had been entirely free from all known growth-retarding factors, so that standards of presumably normal fetal growth, as seen in newborn infants, could be constructed. Even with approximately 6000 mothers, we could not find enough control mothers, i.e., free from all known growth-retarding influences in their pregnancies, to construct standards of normal fetal growth for premature infants.

We have not tried to review all the literature on fetal growth in humans. Our approach to this fairly complex problem with its large number of known growth-retarding factors differed considerably from that of most previous investigators in the manner and methods by which presumably normally grown newborn infants were selected and the manner and methods by which single and multiple growth-retarding factors were considered. Furthermore, we differed considerably in the way in which we determined pregnancy outcome for fetuses. Instead of using birth weight in relation to gestational age as the determinant of fetal growth, we have broadened our objectives to include premature births, the two main types of fetal growth retardation in full-term infants and the important group of infants known as low birth weight infants (< 2500 gm).

The limitations of the study should be recognized. The diagnosis of the symmetrically undergrown fetus (labeled by us as short-for-dates) depended on knowing the gestational age of the fetus and there obviously was some error involved in calculating gestational age, just as there is in diagnosing the newborn infant who has a low birth weight for gestational age. It was difficult in some infants to determine if their births had been premature (< 37 completed weeks of gestation) or if they were undergrown full-term infants, because the duration of pregnancy might be unknown or uncertain and because the physical signs of maturation in the newborn infant might have developed unevenly or even have been retarded by the same factors that retarded somatic growth. For these reasons, we included in our data the category of newborn infants known as low birth weight (< 2500 gm) infants; their diagnosis rested solely on their birth weights. All infants in this study were weighed almost always within the first half hour after their births on highly reliable scales.

1 / Objectives

MANY INVESTIGATORS in the past half century have studied fetal growth in humans as though fetuses were a breed apart from other growing members of the human family. They relied heavily on weights obtained at birth to determine how well or poorly fetuses grew and showed a great reluctance to use external body measurements in their evaluations of fetal growth. No investigator or clinician would characterize growth in older infants and children simply on the basis of body weight in relation to age. All postnatal growth charts provide for measurements of height, weight and head circumference, presumably as being basic determinants of postnatal growth. Failure to use measurements of crown-heel length at birth as a vital part of evaluating fetal growth has created an impasse in the diagnosis of fetal growth retardation (FGR) among some investigators. They have defined FGR in terms of a low birth weight in relation to fetal age, using such terms as small for gestational age (SGA) or small-for-dates (SFD) to describe such infants. These definitions are helpful so far as they go, but they do not go far enough. SGA and SFD do not distinguish between the two main types of FGR, and by using a low cutoff weight of 2500 or 2600 gm or some arbitrarily selected percentile of birth weight, investigators have failed to diagnose FGR in infants whose birth weights happen to be above these low birth weights. The same criticism applies to the study of overgrown fetuses; birth weight in relation to gestational age does not differentiate between the two main types of fetal overgrowth.

Our objectives in writing this text were several: to expand the number of atypical fetal growth patterns presently being recognized; to present for the first time anthropometric data on newborn infants who were free from all known growth-retarding influences in utero, so far as one could tell from examining the infants at birth and from reviewing their mothers' medical and

1

obstetric records and from personal interviews with the mothers; to use body measurements of newborn infants obtained with specific techniques by a single person (HCM) to construct standards of presumably normal fetal growth for purposes of comparisons with newborn infants with atypical fetal growth patterns and to describe the causes and consequences of atypical fetal growth.

There are two main types of FGR, evidently first described by Gruenwald and later confirmed by other investigators.[1-4] In the first type, the infant has a normal crown-heel length for fetal age but is deficient in subcutaneous fat and possibly to some extent in skeletal muscle. Naeye[5] observed that such infants also had reduced weights of their livers, spleens, adrenals and thymus glands. In the second type, the infant is symmetrically small at birth in external body dimensions for gestational age but not necessarily underweight for height. Some full-term infants who are symmetrically small for their gestational ages are also lean and deficient in subcutaneous fat and thus have both types of FGR. Gruenwald suggested that the first type occurred late in pregnancy and that the second type had its origins much earlier in pregnancy. No one to date has disagreed with his suggestion that these two types of FGR differ in their pathogenesis.

Not only do these two types of FGR probably differ in their pathogenesis but they also differ in their postnatal courses.[6] Infants who are long and lean at birth tend to have large appetites and to accelerate their weight gains and thus catch up in weight to normal control* infants within 3–6 months of their births. On the other hand, infants who are symmetrically small for their gestational ages at birth tend to have ordinary appetites; some of them remain short in stature despite satisfactory growth rates in height. The probable differences in pathogenesis and the specific differences in postnatal courses clearly indicate the need to distinguish between these two types of FGR. If these two types of FGR are diagnosed, as they should be, by appropriate techniques and not by a low birth weight for gestational age, it be-

---

*The word *control* has been used throughout this text to designate mothers and infants of mothers who to our knowledge had none of the growth-retarding factors in their pregnancies listed in Table 3–1. It is not meant to indicate that these mothers or their infants constituted a control group in the formal meaning of the word.

comes apparent that there are more undergrown fetuses than previously recognized.[7, 8] The use solely of a low birth weight for gestational age, which usually is less than 2500 or 2600 gm, has prevented infants with heavier birth weights from being diagnosed under the term FGR.

The heavy reliance on birth weight alone to diagnose FGR relates to the ease and accuracy of its measurement and to the recognized correlation between birth weight and body size. However, the correlation between weight and size is not a good one. We previously demonstrated that infants of the same body length, sex, race and gestational age varied by as much as 1100 gm in their birth weights.[9] Such wide variations in birth weights relate to differences in soft tissue mass, including fat, skeletal muscle and some viscera, and preclude birth weight from being in itself a highly valid measure of body size.

There are two types of fetal overgrowth. In one type, the infant is of normal size but is obese. In the other type, the infant has large body dimensions for gestational age but is not obese. The two types of FGR and the two types of fetal overgrowth can be diagnosed by measuring external body dimensions and by calculating either weight-height ratios or ponderal indices. Inspection and palpation of newborn infants provides an excellent beginning in the diagnosis of lean and obese infants; measurements of skin fold thickness at appropriate sites are helpful adjuncts. Symmetrically small and large infants can be diagnosed by comparing their external body dimensions with those of control infants.

Investigators have been reluctant to use measurements of crown-heel length in diagnosing small and large infants, because they probably deemed such measurements to be unreliable. A recent publication of the United States government describes and illustrates a method for measuring crown-heel lengths of infants. The publication states that "Measurement of length is difficult and should not be attempted unless satisfactory equipment and two trained examiners are available. In many instances, it will not be practical to measure length routinely."[10] Some techniques for measuring body length of infants are unreliable and should be abandoned. The problem in measuring infants' lengths is overcoming the flexed position of their legs. This problem can be circumvented by making use of the tonic-neck reflex to help overcome their flexed positions. The infant is placed in a shallow box against the far side in order to maintain a straight position for head, neck and back. The head is turned toward the examiner and fixed against the top side of the box with the right hand; the left hand fixes the right leg in a straight position without tilting the pelvis (Fig. 1–1). Having fixed the head and right leg and foot, the right hand is released to bring up a movable panel to the sole of the right foot. The length can be read off directly on a centimeter rule fastened in position to the box. This method has been previously published along with tests of its reliability.[9] It is a simple method that with a little practice can be carried out by a single person. The crown-heel length of infants in incubators and in some ventilators can be measured by using a stiff metal rod of appropriate length with a fixed head-plate and a sliding footplate. Davies and Holding[11] have described a more elaborate method, utilizing a neonatometer that requires 2 persons to operate. They also have published data on its reliability. Other methods of measuring body length have been used, but in no instance have we seen results of tests of their reliability. Some of the published studies on fetal growth have not even provided the reader with the method used in mea-

Fig. 1–1. – Method for measuring body length, using tonic-neck reflex to overcome flexion of leg. (Reproduced, with permission, from Pediatrics 48(4):511. Copyright American Academy of Pediatrics, 1971.)

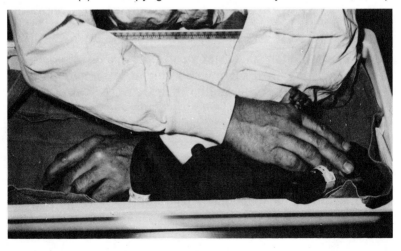

suring body length. Most other measurements of external body dimensions can be easily and reliably made, with the exception of crown-rump length. Reliability of crown-rump measurements in newborn infants is poor, because in many infants the amount of subcutaneous fat on the buttocks varies widely and interferes with an accurate measurement of linear skeletal size.

There are many different atypical patterns of fetal growth. In this text, consideration is given to six atypical patterns. In addition to the four atypical patterns of fetal undergrowth and overgrowth described above there are disproportionate growth and congenital malformations. Congenital malformations are discussed in Chapter 20 in connection with short stature and the causes of the latter. Disproportionate growth in this text involves disproportion between head size and body length. Usually there is a direct proportion between growth in head circumference and crown-heel length during the fetal period. Little attention has been given to this observation. Head size at birth is directly proportional to crown-heel length, but not in all infants. In perhaps 5–10% of infants, the head is large or small in proportion to a normal body length or the latter is short or long in proportion to a normal head circumference. The clinical significance of these disproportions has not been investigated. The importance of disproportionate growth at present lies in its implications for sonographers who attempt to estimate gestational age and body size and weight by measuring biparietal diameters of fetal heads. Sonographers are bound to encounter some fetuses with large heads and short bodies and other fetuses with small heads and long bodies.

A major objective of this text is the preparation of standards based on measurements of newborn infants who have been unencumbered by known growth-retarding influences in utero, so far as could be determined from review of their mothers' medical and obstetric histories and from examination of the infants. Previously published standards have not attempted to exclude all infants with a potential fetal growth-retarding factor (see Chap. 4). By excluding all infants with known growth-retarding conditions from the standard group, a better opportunity is afforded in diagnosing excessive fetal undergrowth and overgrowth and in elucidating their causes.

Much has been written about low birth weight (LBW) infants

(< 2500 gm). They constitute a heterogeneous group, including premature infants (< 37 completed weeks of gestation) and at least the two main types of FGR seen in infants of 37 weeks or more. Their importance as a group depends on two factors. They are easily diagnosed by the simple process of weighing them and they provide, as a group, a good indication of the degree of progress being made in prenatal care of mothers and their fetuses.[12] It is generally recognized that any substantial reduction in their numbers will alleviate pressures on intensive care units for ill newborn infants, decrease the number of crib deaths occurring in the early postnatal months,[13] lower infant mortality and diminish long-term morbidity arising from premature birth and severe fetal growth retardation. In the present text, frequent reference is made to this important group of infants in order to demonstrate as specifically as possible the factors responsible for their births.

Last and far from least of the purposes in writing this text is to call attention to the fact that factors leading to FGR are also likely to be associated with premature birth. Data are presented throughout the text that amply support this statement. Prevention of premature births has not been given the high priority it deserves in perinatal research.

REFERENCES
1. Gruenwald, P.: Chronic fetal distress and placental insufficiency, Biol. Neonate 5:215, 1963.
2. Omsted, M., and Taylor, M. E.: The postnatal growth of children who were small-for-dates or large-for-dates at birth, Dev. Med. Child Neurol. 13:421, 1971.
3. Dubowitz, V.: The infant of inappropriate size. Size at birth, Ciba Foundation Symposium, pp. 47–82, 1971.
4. Cook, L. N.: Intrauterine and extrauterine recognition and management of deviant fetal growth, Pediatr. Clin. North Am. 24:431, 1977.
5. Naeye, R. L.: Malnutrition, probable cause of fetal growth retardation, Arch. Pathol. 70:284, 1965.
6. Holmes, G. E., Miller, H. C., Hassanein, K., Lansky, S. B., and Goggin, J. E.: Postnatal somatic growth in infants with atypical fetal growth patterns, Am. J. Dis. Child. 131:1078, 1977.
7. Miller, H. C., and Hassanein, K.: Fetal malnutrition in white newborn infants: Maternal factors, Pediatrics 52:504, 1973.
8. Miller, H. C., and Hassanein, K.: Maternal factors in "fetally malnourished" black newborn infants, Am. J. Obstet. Gynecol. 118:62, 1974.
9. Miller, H. C., and Hassanein, K.: Diagnosis of impaired fetal growth in newborn infants, Pediatrics 48:511, 1971.

10. Fomon, S. J.: Nutritional Disorders of Children. U.S. Department of Health, Education, and Welfare, Public Health Service. DHEW Publication No. (HSA) 76-5612, 1976.
11. Davies, D. P., and Holding, R. E.: Neonatometer: A new infant length measurer, Arch. Dis. Child. 47:938, 1972.
12. Miller, H. C., Hassanein, K., and Hensleigh, P.: Maternal factors in the incidences of low birth weight infants among black and white mothers, Pediatr. Res. 12:1016, 1978.
13. Vaughan, V. C., and McKay, R. J.: *Nelson's Textbook of Pediatrics* (10th ed.; Philadelphia: W. B. Saunders Company, 1975), p. 1647.

2 / Metabolic and Nutritional Factors

HUMAN FETAL GROWTH results from an interplay of maternal, fetal and placental factors. The nutritional supply to the fetus provided by the uteroplacental circulation, the transfer of substrate across the placenta, the fetal endocrine milieu and the expression of the fetal genome are important in fetal ontogeny. This chapter summarizes the numerous factors already identified as controlling growth potential in the human fetus. Substantial contributions to the understanding of basic interrelationships have been derived from animal studies. Experiments of nature and other circumstances that are unfavorable to normal fetal growth in man have provided insights into the many factors that control feto-maternal interactions and alter fetal growth in humans.

Cellular and organ growth.—The incremental increase in body mass that constitutes fetal growth needs to be considered at the cellular, tissue, organ and organismic levels. The rate of growth is mainly determined by the rate of net protein synthesis. Growth ceases when anabolic and catabolic rates reach equilibrium. Winick[1] has suggested that fetal growth is a homogeneous process, inasmuch as accretion of net protein has been demonstrated to be linear in all organs in utero.

Enesco and LeBlond[2] assumed diploid constancy of each developing human cell and evaluated organ growth by determining the increase in cell number, measured by the total content of DNA in the organ, and the increase in cell size, measured by the weight or protein content of the organ per unit of DNA. In the human diploid nucleus, the amount of DNA per cell is fixed at 6.0 picograms of DNA per cell nucleus.[3] An increase in DNA thus represents growth by mitotic activity. No increase in DNA per incremental increase in total tissue or in the protein content

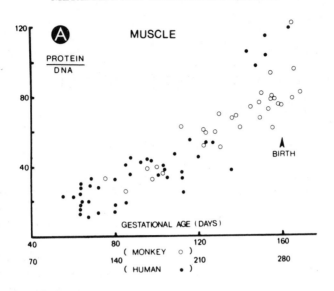

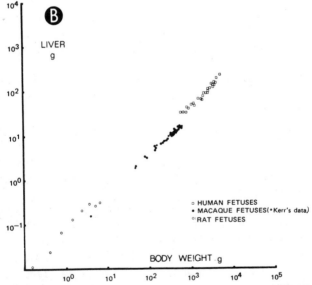

Fig. 2–1.—A, protein/DNA in skeletal muscle in the fetal human and macaque. The gestational age for the monkey has been compared on an equivalent scale for comparison. (With permission of D. Cheek.) **B,** the growth of the liver relative to the body as a whole for man, macaque and the rat during fetal life. (With permission of D. Cheek.) *(Continued)*

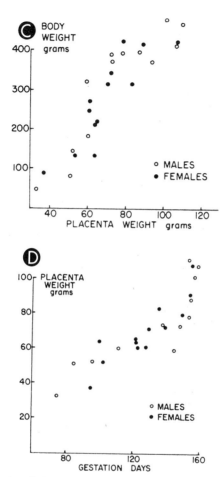

Fig. 2–1 (cont.). — **C,** increase of macaque placental weight compared to increase in fetal body weight. **D,** increase in macaque placental weight as a function of gestational age. (From Cheek, D. B. [ed.]:*Fetal and Postnatal Cellular Growth* [New York: John Wiley & Sons, Inc., 1975]. Reprinted by permission of the publisher and D. Cheek.)

of the organ represents growth by enlargement of cells already in existence. Using this technique, Winick[4] quantified growth in terms of cellular and organ growth in several species, including the human, and described three distinct phases of growth. During normal growth, total DNA content of organs (cell number) increases linearly and then decelerates, reaching its maximum long before organ size, as measured by net protein synthesis, reaches its maximum. From this pattern of cellular DNA and protein synthesis, Winick described three phases of growth.

Phase 1. *Hyperplasia* — proportional increase in weight, protein and DNA content of tissues.

Phase 2. *Hyperplasia and concomitant hypertrophy* — increase in DNA content slower than the increases in protein and weight of tissues.

Phase 3. *Hypertrophy* — no further increase in DNA content but continued increase in weight and protein content of tissues.

Winick and Noble[5] demonstrated that undernutrition during hyperplastic growth curtailed the rate of cell division and could result, if the undernutrition was prolonged, in an organ with a permanently reduced cell number. The same degrees of nutrition imposed during the hypertrophic phase retarded the expected increase in cell size. This latter insult was reversible on institution of proper nutrition. Exhaustive studies in the rat and selective postnatal studies in human infants with varying degrees of malnutrition revealed similar growth patterns in a variety of organs.[6-8] Growth of the human placenta follows the same patterns as other organs.[9] Dobbing and Sands[10] evaluated the growth of the human brain and demonstrated peaks of DNA synthesis occurring at 26 weeks' gestation and again shortly after birth. Cheek[11] has published extensively on differential organ growth in the fetal rhesus monkey. Graphic representation of his findings are summarized in Figure 2–1, A to 2–1, D. Skeletal muscle of the human fetus constitutes 25–50% of body weight during the last half of gestation and serves as a useful model for studying growth and cellular functional differentiation.[12] During this period, nuclear number, calculated from increases in number of muscle cells, increased from 5×10^9 to 40×10^9 and muscle protein/DNA increased 2.6-fold, indicating that both hyperplasia and hypertrophy of muscle cells were occurring.[13] Dubowitz[14] defined the developmental histochemistry of fetal skeletal muscle as related to maturation. Until the end of the first half of gestation, no clear division exists between fetal muscle types. Sheaths have not developed around muscle fiber groups and fiber size is variable. Histochemically, the muscle fibers are similar. From the 20th to 26th weeks, fetal muscle separates into types I and II fibers. From 30 weeks to term, development of muscle fiber corresponds to more mature or adult-type configurations with equal numbers of I and II fiber types. Although Dubowitz was unable to observe differences in muscle growth in fetuses with intrauterine growth retardation, Cheek and Hill[12] found differences in muscle growth in infants suffering from postnatal marasmus and kwashiorkor. In these latter infants, cell fiber length was reduced, cell size was small and RNA, zinc and magnesium were low in relation to DNA content. Insulin levels were low, probably because of diminished secretion of insulin in utero. These older malnourished infants were similar to the long, lean malnourished fetuses described by Naeye[15] and Miller.[16] This model of fetal muscle growth serves to conceptualize the belief that growth can be differentiated from maturation of organ function; the latter depends on the emergence of sequential enzymatic pathways that are affected by a host of hormones affecting the fetal genome.

Placental regulation. — Placental growth is critical for fetal growth. Restriction of placental and fetal growth has been observed when maternal nutrition has been insufficient.[17, 18] A placenta with a massive infarction is shown in Figure 2–2, A and B. It is obvious that growth would be altered in a fetus surviving so massive an infarction, because of the reduced placental area for perfusion and substrate transfer. Normal placentas increase in size almost linearly up to 36 weeks. Placental growth is influenced by human placental lactogen (hPL) and human chorionic gonadotropin (HCG). Low levels of hPL, secreted by the syncytiotrophoblasts, in the maternal serum have been associated with fetal growth retardation. The hPL has been detected as early as 5 weeks of gestation and increases during pregnancy to a peak at about 36 weeks. It is hypothesized that hPL serves to regulate delivery of maternal substrate to the fetus. Spellacy[19] correlated fetal weight, placental weight and maternal levels of hPL during the last month of pregnancy. Low or falling hPL levels were found to be associated with placental insufficiency, fetal distress or fetal demise. It is of considerable interest that markedly elevated levels of hPL have been found in maternal sera in twin pregnancies. HCG, derived from the corpus luteum of pregnancy, is produced early in pregnancy. High levels are reached dur-

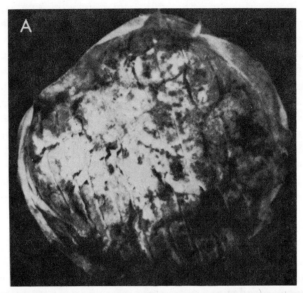

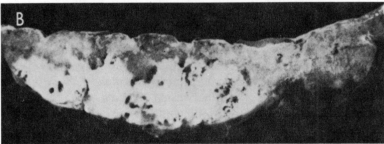

Fig. 2–2.—**A,** massive infarction of the placenta as illustrated by the white, firm and well-defined lesions in the decidua. **B,** on the sagittal cut surface the extent of the placental infarct is obvious. It is evident that a substantial portion of the exchange area has been injured, with destruction of villi and adjacent septal tissue. Diminished perfusion and a reduction in substrate transfer to the fetus results. (Courtesy of Dr. Kurt Benirschke.)

ing the first trimester of gestation. HCG appears to bestow maternal immunologic tolerance on the fetus. Thomson[20] observed a significant correlation between placental weight and infant birth weight. He found that not all small-for-dates infants had proportionally smaller placentas. Scott and Usher[21] as well as Younoszai and Haworth[22] detected a proportionate reduction in both fetal and placental weights in pregnancies ending with infants who were small for gestational ages. When the placenta reached a weight of about 300 gm or when fetal weight approximated 2.3 kg at about 36 weeks, the DNA content of the placenta was fixed. Thus, during the last month of gestation, the rapidly growing fetus is nourished by an organ of maximal cellular composition. Studies of poor Indian and Guatemalan gravidas showed marked differences in the cellular composition of placentas, depending on whether or not the infants were normal or small-for-dates.[23] Winick *et al.*[24] and Iyengar[25] demonstrated a significant reduction in cell number, protein, glycogen and alkaline phosphatase of placentas when mothers were delivered of small-for-dates infants. Placental glycogen decreases with advancing gestation and placental alkaline phosphatase increases toward term. Numerous comparisons have been made between placentas associated with normally grown fetuses and those with intrauterine growth failure. Qualitative morphologic differences in the placentas from malnourished fetuses are characterized by an umbilical cord of small caliber with reduced spirals, diminished circumference and an over-all reduction in placental thickness.[26] Animal models have established that diminished availability of maternal substrates from either undernutrition or diminished uterine blood flow produces these changes in placental morphology. Conversely, large placentas with increased glycogen content are a frequent finding accompanying macrosomic fetuses of diabetic women. Hypercellularity of the latter placentas suggests that fetal hyperinsulinemia promotes placental growth and hyperplasia.

Substrate control over growth.—Glucose is a major maternal substrate utilized by the growing fetus and is transplacentally distributed to the fetal circulation via facilitated transport mechanisms.[27] Liver glycogen stores in the fetus increase dramatically after the 36th week of pregnancy. Glycogen stored during the last month of the third trimester enhances the glycolytic capacity of the fetus during perinatal stress that comes with transient hypoxemia, cessation of umbilical blood flow and neonatal cold stress. Amino acids are also a major nutrient supplied to the fetus and also require an energy-consuming transfer mechanism. The diffusion capacity of the placenta for both glucose and amino

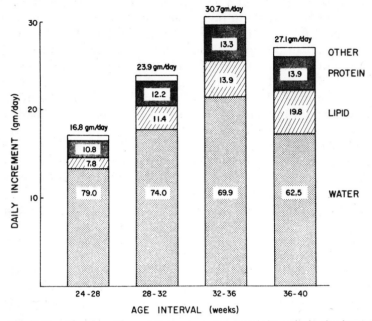

Fig. 2–3.—Composition of the progressive weight gain in the human fetus during the last trimester. Numbers at the top of each bar indicate the mean weight gain/day. (From Growth 40:338, 1976. Reproduced by permission.)

acid increases proportionately with increased fetal growth during pregnancy.[27] The third trimester of gestation in humans is characterized by the deposition of adipose tissue in the fetus. Fetal fat stores provide thermal insulation postnatally and can also be used for caloric needs during extrauterine adaptation. Fatty acid synthetase isozymes provide the prime pathway for the synthesis of long-chain fatty acids. The greatest activity of these enzymes is in the fetal liver and lung.[28] The activity of acetyl-Co A carboxylase, which is the rate-limiting step in fatty acid synthesis, drops in the fetal liver with the onset of feeding postnatally but remains elevated in the lungs throughout the neonatal period.[29] An optimal exchange of oxygen and carbon dioxide by the placenta is essential for providing substrates of glucose and amino acids. Relative deficiencies of oxygen, as experienced at high altitude or in certain maternal diseases and conditions, have adverse effects on fetal growth.[30] The recognized decrement in fetal weight and early delivery associated with maternal smoking probably is an example of impaired oxygen transport through the placenta. Increased levels of carboxyhemoglobin have been found in the fetal circulation in these infants.[31]

The electrolyte and mineral composition of the body of a "reference" (mean of 5 fetuses) fetus[32] compared to maternal serum levels demonstrates a maternal to fetal gradient, yielding a net fetal gain in zinc, copper, iron, manganese and chromium.[32-34] These minerals are important cofactors for lipid and protein synthesis in the developing fetus. Incremental increases in protein, lipids, water and electrolytes during the last trimester are presented in Figure 2–3.

Vitamins serve as important cofactors for fetal growth.[35] Levels of vitamins in fetal cord blood indicate the existence of a maternal to fetal flux for folic acid, B_6, riboflavin, nicotinic acid, pantothenic acid, thiamine, biotin and B_{12}. Only vitamin A and β-carotene levels are higher in maternal than in fetal sera. Low birth weight infants have exhibited significantly lower levels of B_{12}, folate and pantothenate in their sera than infants who had normal birth weights.[36]

Insulin and glucagon. — Recent advances in fetal endocrinology have recorded the many growth-controlling factors that are mediated by multiple hormones throughout gestation. Maternal insulin does not cross the placenta. Release of fetal insulin and glucagon is stimulated by a peptide secreted in the ventrolateral hypothalamic region.[37] Coupled with simultaneous parasympathetic innervation of the fetal pancreas, this neural peptide augments release of insulin and secretion of glucagon. Insulin has been found in fetuses as early as the 8th week and substantial evidence has accumulated that fetal insulin by 8–10 weeks significantly influences biochemical events that regulate the fetal pancreas.[38, 39] Both direct and indirect evidence have demonstrated that fetal beta cells in the human are responsive to the administration of glucose or arginine to mothers.[40] During periods of maternal feeding, fetal glucose levels follow maternal serum glucose levels, although there is a delay in maternal to fetal glucose equilibrium with a slight decrease in fetal levels compared to maternal serum levels. Increased levels of fetal glucose are followed by elevations in fetal insulin, thus promoting the uptake and storage of glucose as glycogen, lipogenesis and the uptake and utilization of amino acids for protein synthesis.

Syndromes characterized by excessive fetal growth have clearly been associated with elevated insulin release. Fetal islet cell tumors (insulinomas) characteristically produce fetal and neonatal macrosomia. Hyperplasia of islets of Langerhans and fetal macrosomia are also found in the Beckwith-Wiedmann syndrome, erythroblastosis and infants of diabetic mothers.

Infants born with diabetes or having pancreatic agenesis are short and light for gestational age. These syndromes are characterized by low or absent levels of fetal insulin.[41] Animal studies, using pancreatectomized fetal lambs or pharmacologic ablation of islet functions in fetal animals, demonstrate striking similarities to fetal insulinopenia and to infants born deficient in fetal insulin.[42] Studies of human fetal glucagon are less conclusive. Fetuses with intrapartum distress and a pH of < 7.2 in blood from scalp capillaries have been reported to have high glucagon levels. Milner and associates[43] reported plasma glucagon levels in umbilical veins to be identical with maternal plasma levels at birth. In their studies, plasma glucagon levels in fetuses did not correlate with either blood glucose or insulin levels. Babies with hemolytic disease of the newborn have been found to have high glucagon levels at birth. Whether these inexplicably high levels of glucagon in infants with erythroblastosis fetalis are the result of prolonged hypoxemia and acidemia in utero is speculative.

Growth hormone.—Concentrations of maternal growth hormone (GH) in maternal serum are low in pregnancy and do not substantially rise during gestation.[44, 45] Maternal GH does not cross the placenta in early pregnancy and cannot be found in the cord sera of newborns. The peak level of GH achieved during the postpartum period in the mother by induced hypoglycemia does not correlate with neonatal birth weight.[46] Infants born to hypophysectomized mothers or to mothers having isolated GH deficiency or acromegaly also appear to be unaffected by perturbations in maternal GH levels.[47, 48]

Fetal growth hormone has been detected in human fetal pituitary tissue culture from 5 weeks of age to late in gestation.[49] Fetal GH increases from 10 to 34 weeks and remains constant during the last 6 weeks of gestation, becoming equal to levels of GH in cord blood. Postnatal levels of GH in sera of newborn infants depend on their gestational ages; premature infants have elevated levels of GH for as long as 2 months after birth, and in term infants GH rises transiently and then remains relatively constant.[50]

Kaplan *et al.*[51] have suggested that GH has little effect on fetal growth. Studies of anencephalic infants and dwarfs suggest that GH has some effect on fetal growth. Honnebier and Swaab[52] and Kittinger[53] reported that birth weights of anencephalic fetuses were significantly less than those of control infants, even after correcting for the missing brain tissue. Shortened body lengths have been reported in infants with familial dwarfism who had high levels of biologically inactive GH.[54] Naeye and Blanc,[55] using quantitative micromorphologic techniques, reported smaller organs (heart, adrenal, liver, lungs, spleens, kidneys) in anencephalic babies and reductions in cell number in the heart, spleen, kidneys and adrenal cortex of these infants. Cheek and Hill[56] suggested that a major role for GH is mitotic regulation during fetal morphogenesis. Naeye and Blanc believe that fetal GH does affect organ growth in the fetus. Additional evidence supporting the latter authors' contention is gained from fetuses suffering spontaneous decapitation.[57-60] Their body weights were consistently low even after correction for the absent heads.[57-60] The regulatory function of GH in fetuses should receive further study.

Thyroid hormone. — Human thyroid tissue is found in fetuses by the third month and thyroxine has been identified in fetal plasma at 15 weeks.[61] The release of thyroxine is dependent on trophic stimulation of TSH by thyroid-releasing hormone (TRH), a tripeptide found in the cerebral cortex, brain stem and cerebellum.[62] In addition to trophic stimulation of the thyroid, TRH also has a role in promoting heat conservation and influencing fetal prolactin secretion. A limited number of athyroid infants have been described as having a significant decrease in body length, a delay in skeletal ossification and reduced neural maturation for a given gestational age and a substantial decrease in fetal ion transport.[63] Similar findings have been reported in rats after ablation of the thyroid soon after birth.[64] Substantial reductions in growth were reported in their kidneys, hearts, livers, muscle and spleens. The focal growth failure in selected tissues was believed to be secondary to specific vulnerabilities in these tissues during the proliferative phase of their growth. Obviously, such findings would be difficult to document in human newborns. However, studies of undiagnosed cretins have confirmed several observations made in subhuman primates and other species.[65] Maternal hyperthyroidism also alters fetal growth in a predictable way. Such infants often show accelerated neurologic maturation and advanced skeletal ossification but have normal birth weights.

Somatomedin.—Somatomedin is a peptide that influences the peripheral action of growth hormone on the proliferation of epiphyseal cartilage and consequently is a potent regulator of fetal growth. Somatomedin levels in the cord plasma and maternal plasma are identical, but these levels are lower than those found in normal nonpregnant females.[66] The comparatively lower somatomedin levels in the fetus and newborn suggest either that fetal tissues are more sensitive to this peptide or that less somatomedin is protein-bound in the human fetus. Infants and young children with kwashiorkor or marasmus have low serum levels of somatomedin in the presence of markedly elevated growth hormone, suggesting that somatomedin is inversely involved in the feedback inhibition of growth hormone.[67] Specific factors producing lowered levels of somatomedin in conditions of inadequate nutrition remain to be identified. Further investigation is needed to determine if fetal malnutrition is associated with reduced levels of somatomedin.

Kidney.—The fetal kidney also has a role in fetal growth. By participating in fetal electrolyte and water homeostasis and contributing to amniotic fluid volume, the kidney exerts both hormonal and environmental constraints on fetal growth. Infants with bilateral renal agenesis (Potter's syndrome) manifest growth retardation and pulmonary hypoplasia.[68] Furthermore, the oligohydramnios resulting from renal dysgenesis and/or urinary obstruction in utero leads to characteristic constraints on fetal growth with shortened and contracted limbs and typical facies. Degradation of fetal insulin occurs in the fetal kidney. Derangements in insulin metabolism, covered earlier in this chapter, profoundly influence fetal growth.

Other constraints.—In addition to the nutritional, placental, genetic and endocrine factors regulating fetal growth there are many factors that retard fetal growth. The latter are discussed in detail in appropriate chapters of this book.

REFERENCES

1. Winick, M.: Fetal malnutrition and growth processes, Hosp. Practice May, 1970, pp. 33–41.
2. Enesco, M., and LeBlond, C. P.: Increase in cell number as a factor in the growth of the organs and tissues of the young male rat, J. Embryol. Exp. Morphol. 10:530, 1962.
3. Mirsky, A. E., and Ris, H.: Variable and constant components of chromosomes, Nature 163:666, 1949.
4. Winick, M.: Cellular changes during placental and fetal growth, Am. J. Obstet. Gynecol. 109:166, 1971.
5. Winick, M., and Noble, A.: Cellular response in rats during malnutrition at various ages, J. Nutr. 89:300, 1966.
6. Brasel, J., and Winick, M.: Differential cellular growth in the organs of hypothyroid rats, Growth 34:197, 1970.
7. Winick, M., Rosso, P., and Waterlow, J.: Cellular growth of cerebrum, cerebellum and brain stem in normal and marasmic children, Exp. Neurol. 26:393, 1970.
8. Winick, W., and Rosso, P.: The effect of severe early malnutrition on cellular growth of human brain, Pediatr. Res. 3:181, 1969.
9. Winick, M., Coscia, A., and Noble, A.: Cellular growth in human placenta. I. Normal placental growth, Pediatrics 39:248, 1967.
10. Dobbing, J., and Sands, J.: Quantitative growth and development of human brain, Arch. Dis. Child. 48:757, 1973.
11. Cheek, D.: *Fetal and Postnatal Cellular Growth* (New York: John Wiley & Sons, 1975), p. 209.
12. Cheek, D. B., and Hill, D. E.: Muscle and liver cell growth: Role of hormones and nutritional factors, Fed. Proc. 29:4, 1503, 1970.
13. Widdowson, E. M., Crabb, D. E., and Milner, R. D. G.: Arch. Dis. Child. 47:652, 1972.
14. Dubowitz, V. D.: Enzyme histochemistry of skeletal muscle, J. Neurol. Neurosurg. Psychiatry 28:516, 1965.
15. Naeye, R. L.: Malnutrition, probable cause of fetal growth retardation, Arch. Pathol. 79:284, 1965.
16. Miller, H. C.: Fetal growth and neonatal mortality, Pediatrics 49:392, 1972.
17. Aherne, W., and Dunnell, M. S.: Morphometry of the human placenta, Br. Med. Bull. 22:5, 1966.
18. Tremblay, P. C., Sybulski, S., and Maugham, C. B.: Role of the placenta in fetal malnutrition, Am. J. Obstet. Gynecol. 91:597, 1965.
19. Spellacy, W. N.: Immunoassay of Human Placental Lactogen, in Wolstenholme, G. W., and Knight, J. (eds.), *Physiological Studies in Normal and Abnormal Pregnancy.* Ciba Foundation (London: Churchill Livingstone, 1972).
20. Thomson, A. M.: The weight of the placenta in relation to birthweight, J. Obstet. Gynecol. Br. Commonw. 76:865, 1969.
21. Scott, K. E., and Usher, R.: Fetal malnutrition, its incidence, causes and effects, Am. J. Obstet. Gynecol. 94:951, 1966.
22. Younoszai, M. K., and Haworth, J. C.: Placental dimensions and

relations in pre-term, term and growth retarded infants, Am. J. Obstet. Gynecol. 103:265, 1969.

23. Dayton, D., Filer, J. L., and Canosa, D.: Cellular changes in the placentas of undernourished mothers in Guatemala, Pediatr. Proc. 28:488, 1969.

24. Winick, M., Velasco, E., and Ross, P.: DNA content of placenta and fetal brain, Proceedings of Pan American Health Organization, Washington, D.C., 1969.

25. Iyengar, L.: Chemical composition of placenta in pregnancies with small-for-dates infants, Am. J. Obstet. Gynecol. 116:66, 1973.

26. McKeown, T., and Record, R. G.: The influence of placental size on foetal growth in man, with special reference to multiple pregnancy, J. Endocrinol. 9:418, 1953.

27. Meschia, G., Battaglia, F. C., and Bruns, P. D.: Theoretical and experimental study of transplacental diffusion, J. Appl. Physiol. 22:1171, 1967.

28. Gross, I., and Warshaw, J. B.: Enzyme activities related to fatty acid synthesis in the developing lung, Pediatr. Res. 8:193, 1974.

29. Warshaw, J. B.: Cellular energy metabolism during fetal development. IV. Fatty acid activation, acetyl transfer and fatty acid oxidation during development of the chick and rat, Dev. Biol. 28:537, 1972.

30. Longo, L. D.: Altitude and Maternal and Infant Capabilities, in Kretchmer, N., and Hasselmeyer, E. (eds.), *Horizons in Perinatal Research* (New York: John Wiley & Sons, 1974), p. 94.

31. Longo, L. D.: Disorders of Placental Transfer, in Assali, N. S., and Brinkman, C. R. (eds.), *Pathophysiology of Gestational Disorders,* Vol. 2 (New York: Academic Press, 1972).

32. Ziegler, E. E., O'Donnell, A. M., Nelson, S. E., and Fomau, S. J.: Body composition of the reference fetus, Growth 40:329, 1976.

33. Henkin, R. I., Schulman, J. D., Schulman, C. D., and Bronzert, D. A.: Changes in total, nondiffusible and diffusible plasma zinc and copper during infancy, J. Pediatr. 82:831, 1973.

34. Lighti, E. L., Almond, C. G., Henzel, J. H., and DeWeese, M. S.: Differences in maternal and fetal plasma zinc levels in sheep and goats, Am. J. Obstet. Gynecol. 106:1242, 1970.

35. Baker, H., Frank, O., Thomson, A., Langer, A., Munves, E., DeAngelis, B., and Kaminetskey, H.: Vitamin profiles of 174 mothers and newborns at parturition, Am. J. Clin. Nutr. 28:59, 1975.

36. Baker, H., Thind, I., Frank, O., DeAngelis, B., Caterini, H., and Louria, D.: Vitamin levels in low birth weight newborn infants and their mothers, Am. J. Obstet. Gynecol. 129:521, 1977.

37. Lockhart-Ewart, R. B., Mok, C., and Martin, J. M.: Neuroendocrine control of insulin secretion, Diabetes 25:96, 1976.

38. Like, A. A., and Orci, L.: Embryogenesis of the human pancreatic islets: A light and electron microscopic study, Diabetes (Supp. 2) 21:511, 1972.

39. Adam, P. A., Teramo, K., Raiha, N., Gitlain, D., and Schwartz, R.:

Human fetal insulin metabolism early in gestation. Response to acute elevation of the fetal glucose concentration and placental transfer of human insulin-I-131, Diabetes 18:409, 1969.

40. Andersson, A., Grill, V., Asplund, K., Berne, C., Agren, A., and Hellerstrom: Functional Maturation of the Pancreatic B-Cell, in Camerini-Davalos, R., and Cole, H. (eds.), *Early Diabetes in Early Life* (New York: Academic Press, 1975), p. 49.
41. Hill, D. E.: Insulin and Fetal Growth, in *Diabetes and Other Endocrine Disorders during Pregnancy and in the Newborn* (New York: Alan R. Liss, Inc., 1976), p. 127.
42. Chez, R. A., Mintz, D. H., Epstein, M. F., Fleischman, A. R., Oakes, G. K., and Hutchinson, D. L.: Glucagon metabolism in nonhuman primate pregnancy, Am. J. Obstet. Gynecol. 120:690, 1974.
43. Milner, R. D. G., Leach, F. N., and Jack, P. B. M.: Reactivity of the Fetal Islet, in Sutherland, H. W. (ed.), *Carbohydrate Metabolism in Pregnancy and in Newborn* (Edinburgh: Churchill Livingstone, 1975), p. 83.
44. Kaplan, S. L., and Grumbach, M. M.: Serum chorionic "growth hormone-prolactin" and serum pituitary growth hormone in mother and fetus at term, J. Clin. Endocrinol. Metab. 25:1370, 1965.
45. Yen, S. S. C., Saimaan, N., and Pearson, O. H.: Growth hormone levels in pregnancy, J. Clin. Endocrinol. Metab. 27:1341, 1967.
46. Gitlin, D., Kumate, J., and Morales, C.: Metabolism and maternofetal transfer of human growth hormone in the pregnant woman at term, J. Clin. Endocrinol. Metab. 25:1599, 1965.
47. Little, B., Smith, O. W., Jesseman, A. G., Selenkow, H. A., Van't Hoff, W., Eglin, J. M., and Moore, F. D.: Hypophysectomy during pregnancy in a patient with cancer of the breast. Case report with hormone studies, J. Clin. Endocrinol. Metab. 18:425, 1958.
48. Rimoin, D. G., Holzman, G. B., Merimee, T. J., Rabinowitz, D., Barnes, A. C., Tyson, J. E. A., and McKusick, V. A.: Lactation in the absence of human growth hormone, J. Clin. Endocrinol. Metab. 28:1183, 1968.
49. Siler-Khodr, T. M., Morgenstern, L. L., and Greenwood, F. C.: Hormone synthesis and release from human fetal adenohypophyses in vitro, J. Clin. Endocrinol. Metab. 39:891, 1974.
50. Cornblath, M., Parker, M. L., Reisner, S. H., Forbes, A. E., and Daughaday, W. H.: Secretion and metabolism of growth hormone in premature and full-term infants, J. Clin. Endocrinol. Metab. 24:209, 1965.
51. Kaplan, S. L., Grumbach, M. M., and Shepard, T. H.: The ontogenesis of human fetal hormones. I. Growth hormone and insulin, J. Clin. Invest. 51:3080, 1972.
52. Honnebier, W. J., and Swaab, D. F.: The influence of anencephaly upon intrauterine growth of fetus and placenta and upon gestation length, J. Obstet. Gynaecol. Br. Commonw. 80:577, 1973.
53. Kittinger, G. W.: *Endocrine Regulation of Fetal Development and its Relation to Parturition in the Rhesus Monkey in the Fetus at*

Birth. Ciba Foundation Symposium 47 (Amsterdam: Elsevier, 1977), p. 235.

54. Laron, Z., Karp, M., Pertzelan, A., Kauli, R., Keret, R., and Doron, M.: The Syndrome of Familial Dwarfism and High Plasma Immunoreactive Human Growth Hormone (IR-HGH), in Pecile, A., and Miller, E. E. (eds.), *Growth and Growth Hormone* (Amsterdam: Excerpta Medica, 1972), p. 458.

55. Naeye, R., and Blanc, W. A.: Organ and body growth in anencephaly. A quantitative morphological study, Arch. Pathol. 91:140, 1971.

56. Cheek, D. B., and Hill, D. E.: Muscle and liver cell growth: Role of hormones and nutritional factors, Fed. Proc. 29:1503, 1970.

57. Kloppner, K.: Menschliches Zwischenhirn-, Mittelhirn- und Ruckenmarkswesen, Arch. Gynaekol. 177:82, 1950.

58. Ehrhardt, L.: Seltene Spontan Amputation Durch Amnion-strang, Zentralbl. Gynaekol. 78:1509, 1956.

59. Benesova, D.: Congenital total defect of the head: Acephalic, Acta Univ. Carol. (Med.) Praha 8:869, 1960.

60. Swinburne, L. M.: Spontaneous intrauterine decapitation, Arch. Dis. Child. 42:636, 1967.

61. Fisher, D. A.: Thyroid Function in the Fetus, in Fisher, D. A., and Burrow, G. N. (eds.), *Perinatal Thyroid Physiology and Disease* (New York: Raven Press, 1975), p. 21.

62. Higgins, G. C.: Adrenocortical related maturational events in the fetus, Am. J. Obstet. Gynecol. 126:931, 1976.

63. Cheek, D., Graystone, J., and Niall, M.: Factors controlling fetal growth, Clin. Obstet. Gynecol. 40:925, 1977.

64. Thorburn, G. C.: Role of Thyroid and Kidneys in Fetal Growth, in *Size at Birth*. Ciba Foundation Symposium (Amsterdam: Elsevier, North-Holland, 1974), p. 185.

65. Kerr, G. R., Tyson, I. B., Allen, J., Wallace, J. H., and Scheffler, G.: Deficiency of thyroid hormone and development of the fetal rhesus monkey, Biol. Neonate 2:282, 1972.

66. Hintz, R. L., Seeds, J. M., and Johnsonbaugh, R. E.: Somatomedin and growth hormone in the newborn, Am. J. Dis. Child. 131:1249, 1977.

67. Hintz, R. L., Suskind, R., Amatayakul, K., and Thanagkul, O.: Plasma somatomedin and growth hormone values in child with protein calorie malnutrition, J. Pediatr. 92:153, 1977.

68. Potter, E., and Craig, J. M.: Kidneys, Ureters, Urinary Bladder and Urethra, in *Pathology of the Fetus and the Infant* (3d ed.; Chicago: Year Book Medical Publishers, Inc., 1975), p. 453.

3 / Abnormal Factors Affecting Fetal Growth

FETAL GROWTH IN HUMANS is affected by a host of factors. Some of these factors, including maternal parity, race and height and gestational age and sex of the infant, play a role in all pregnancies. Such factors are considered basic to all pregnancies and are discussed in detail in Chapter 4. Other factors affecting fetal growth appear only in some pregnancies and should be considered abnormal or unusual and not routine factors.

Most of the abnormal factors are of the growth-retarding type and their number is large. In order to simplify the problem of dealing with so large a number of factors, they have been grouped in Table 3–1 under four appropriate headings. The four groups include fetal factors, medical complications of pregnancy, maternal behavioral conditions associated with pregnancy and environmental factors. The feature that distinguishes behavioral conditions of pregnancy in group III, Table 3–1, from the other three groups is the matter of maternal choice, which is present to some degree in each of the seven behavioral conditions. Women adopting any of these seven maternal conditions do have the opportunity of making a choice. Physicians and society in general may warn against adopting these behavioral conditions, but women are in a position to act independently of their warnings, with the exception that in some undeveloped countries, the problem of being underweight for height at conception can be attributed to an inadequate supply of essential foods. The importance of maternal choice as the distinguishing feature of the seven conditions in group III is illustrated in Chapter 5, showing that women in poor socioeconomic circumstances adopt these seven conditions with significantly greater frequency than women living under better conditions. The importance of placing these seven conditions in a separate group from all other factors

TABLE 3-1.—ABNORMAL FACTORS ASSOCIATED
WITH FETAL GROWTH RETARDATION

I. Fetal factors	Intrauterine infections
	Chromosomal aberrations
	Congenital malformations
	Inborn errors of metabolism
	Multiple births
II. Medical complications of pregnancy	Acute or chronic hypertension
	Preeclampsia
	Severe vaginal bleeding (third trimester)
	Severe chronic disease involving heart, liver, lungs, kidneys, gastrointestinal tract, thyroid or adrenal glands
	Disseminated lupus erythematosus
	Sarcoidosis
	Severe chronic infections
	Anemia (< 10 gm/dl)
	Leukemia
	Malignant solid tumors
	Large ovarian cysts
	Multiple large fibroids of uterus
	Continuous medication with corticoids, immunosuppressive, teratogenic or growth-retarding drugs
	Abnormalities of uterus, placenta or umbilical cord
	Polyhydramnios
	Oligohydramnios
III. Selected maternal behavioral conditions associated with pregnancy	1. Abnormally low prepregnancy weight for height
	2. Low maternal weight gain in pregnancy
	3. Lack of any prenatal care
	4. Delivery before seventeenth birthday
	5. Delivery after thirty-fifth birthday
	6. Cigarette smoking during pregnancy
	7. Use of addicting drugs or large amounts of alcohol during pregnancy
IV. Environmental factors	High altitude
	Exposure to toxic substances

is also demonstrated by data in Chapter 5, showing that irrespective of socioeconomic status, the adoption of these conditions carries an added risk for the fetus.

Certain factors that have been associated with retarded fetal growth were omitted from Table 3-1. Reasons for omitting them need to be presented. An important omission is maternal dietary insufficiency, which in itself includes several factors that might make fetal growth less than optimal, such as insufficient calories, protein, essential amino acids, minerals and vitamins. Jacobson[1] recently has reviewed the difficulties in evaluating maternal dietary intakes during pregnancy in American women. He expresses the hope that new techniques, such as computer programming of food intake and use of ultrasound techniques to determine the nutritional status of mothers, may bring about a breakthrough in evaluating maternal nutrition and fetal growth. In the meantime, in connection with data presented in this text, it was hoped that determination of maternal weight gains, especially of poor weight gains during the second and third trimesters, might in part fill the gap created by the omission of dietary factors. Studies by previous investigators testify to the importance of maternal nutrition in fetal growth.[2-6] But no one should underrate the difficulties encountered when one attempts to take into account the many dietary components as well as all other fetal growth-retarding factors.

Socioeconomic factors were also omitted from Table 3–1. It is well known that underprivileged women have more low birth weight infants than gravidas in the upper socioeconomic groups. It is interesting that attempts to identify specific social and economic factors that affect fetal growth adversely have been singularly unsuccessful.[7-9] There is evidence presented in Chapter 5 to show that socioeconomic factors probably are not of primary but may be of secondary importance. Significant differences were not observed in mean birth weights of infants born at The University of Kansas Medical Center to women in different socioeconomic circumstances, provided that they and their infants avoided all the conditions listed in Table 3–1. Data also show that the seven maternal conditions listed in Table 3–1, such as cigarette smoking, and so on, appeared to be primary factors in the poor pregnancy outcome for fetuses in the various socioeconomic groups.

Much has been made of the observation that the birth weight of a later-born infant tends to approximate the birth weights of previously born siblings. Some mothers have a succession of low birth weight infants (< 2500 gm). This repetition of low birth weight infants has been included in some lists as a fetal growth-retarding factor, although without any explanation as to what might have produced a succession of low birth weight infants. A high percentage of these mothers delivered at The University of

Kansas Medical Center were smoking cigarettes during pregnancy and were involved with other unfavorable behavioral conditions listed in Table 3–1. Consequently, they have not been placed in a separate and special group in Table 3–1.

Some studies have included psychiatric disorders in the list of fetal growth-retarding factors. Women with psychosis and lesser emotional disturbances delivered at The University of Kansas Medical Center have had growth-retarded fetuses, but most of these mothers were involved with one or more other growth-retarding factors listed in Table 3–1. The small group who had no other growth-retarding factors is presented in Table 14–1.

Many infants born to mothers with growth-retarding factors in their pregnancies have birth weights, head sizes and body lengths that are within normal ranges for their gestational ages. The fact that their measurements are within the normal range does not mean that they had optimal fetal growth.

If fetuses and newborn infants are to be considered as normally grown in utero and are to be used for control purposes in studies of fetal growth, they and their mothers should be free from all identifiable growth-retarding factors. This method of selecting fetuses and infants for a control group, to which all other fetuses and infants can be compared, has not been used in any of the published data on fetal growth (see Chap. 4).

An important aspect of fetal growth that has not received enough attention is the occurrence of multiple adverse factors in a single pregnancy. The incidence of gravidas with multiple

TABLE 3–2.—INCIDENCE OF LOW BIRTH
WEIGHT (LBW) INFANTS (< 2500 GM)
ACCORDING TO NUMBER OF BEHAVIORAL
CONDITIONS* PRESENT PER PREGNANCY
AMONG WHITE MOTHERS

NO. OF INDEPENDENT VARIABLES PRESENT PER PREGNANCY	MOTHERS	LBW INFANTS	
	No.	No.	%
0	624	6	1.0
1	506	34	6.7
2	168	17	10.1
≥ 3	45	13	28.9

*Behavioral conditions were those listed in group III, Table 3–1.

growth-retarding factors in their pregnancies has been surprisingly high among women delivered at The University of Kansas Medical Center.[10] Pregnancy outcome with respect to the fetus was significantly worse if multiple growth-retarding factors were present. Data in Table 3–2 show that the per cent incidence of low birth weight (LBW) infants (< 2500 gm) rose significantly from 1.0% among mothers with no known growth-retarding factors to 28.9% among women with three or more of the seven behavioral conditions listed in Table 3–1. Using the method of least squares, the regression line of per cent LBW infants on the number of behavioral conditions is fitted. The regression coefficient is 7.80, which is statistically significant from zero ($p < 0.01$). None of the women had medical complications of pregnancy and none of the infants had any of the fetal conditions listed in Table 3–1.

The number of abnormal factors that are known to be associated with excessive stimulation of fetal growth is small. Diabetes mellitus, gestational diabetes and the prediabetic state are the main conditions leading to fetal overgrowth. The possible roles of maternal obesity and of excessive weight gains in pregnancy in overstimulation of fetal growth are discussed in appropriate chapters in this text.

In the chapters that follow, emphasis has been placed on differences in pregnancy outcome among women with no known fetal growth-retarding factors, as listed in Table 3–1, in their pregnancies and women with one or more of the seven behavioral conditions listed there. These differences are important, because they demonstrate that pregnancy outcome was excellent in the first group of women and comparatively poor in the second group. Less attention has been given to pregnancy outcome among women with medical complications of pregnancy. Pregnancy outcome in this group was uniformly poor because of the very high incidence of premature births and of low birth weight (LBW) infants. The incidence of LBW infants in this group was about 20% irrespective of socioeconomic circumstances. Improvement in pregnancy outcome among women with medical complications of pregnancy depends on the skills of physicians and advances in medical science. Emphasis in this text was purposely placed on pregnancy outcome among women with behavioral conditions, because behavior can be modified and, if successfully so, might bring about a marked improvement in perinatal risk for fetuses and newborn infants and improvement in long-term growth, development and survival of many infants.

REFERENCES

1. Jacobson, H. N.: Current concepts in nutrition. Diet in pregnancy, N. Engl. J. Med. 297:1051, 1977.
2. Ebbs, J.: The influence of prenatal diet on the mother and child, J. Nutr. 22:515, 1941.
3. Burke, B. S., Beal, V. A., Kirkwood, B., and Stuart, H. C.: The influence of nutrition during pregnancy upon the condition of the infant at birth, J. Nutr. 26:569, 1943.
4. Smith, C. A.: Effects of maternal undernutrition upon the newborn infant in Holland (1944–45), J. Pediatr. 30:229, 1947.
5. Antonov, A. N.: Children born during the siege of Leningrad in 1942, J. Pediatr. 30:250, 1947.
6. Lechtig, A., Delgado, H., Lasky, R. E., Klein, R. E., Engle, P. L., Yarbrough, C., and Habicht, J. P.: Maternal nutrition and fetal growth in developing societies, Am. J. Dis. Child. 129:434, 1975.
7. Naylor, A. F., and Myrianthopoulos, N. C.: The relation of ethnic and selected socio-economic factors to human birth weight, Ann. Hum. Genet. 31:71, 1967.
8. Comstock, G. W., Shah, F. K., Meyer, M. D., and Abbey, H.: Low birth weight and neonatal mortality rate related to maternal smoking and socioeconomic status, Am. J. Obstet. Gynecol. 111:53, 1971.
9. Morris, N. M., Udry, J. R., and Chase, C. L.: Reduction of low birth weight birth rates by the prevention of unwanted pregnancies, Am. J. Public Health 63:935, 1973.
10. Miller, H. C., Hassanein, K., and Hensleigh, P.: Effects of behavioral and medical variables on fetal growth retardation, Am. J. Obstet. Gynecol. 127:643, 1977.

4 / Anthropometric Data on White Control Infants

SEVERAL BASIC FACTORS have to be considered in evaluating fetal growth in a normal, uncomplicated pregnancy. These are the race, age, height, habitus (weight for height) and parity of the mother and the sex and gestational age of the fetus. These factors affect crown-heel length, head size, habitus and weight of the fetus in different degrees, depending on the factor and the parameter involved. All these factors taken together would appear to make the evaluation of fetal somatic growth a complex matter. The evaluation procedure can be made less complicated by determining its objectives and their relative importance. The primary objectives in the fetus and newborn infant are the same as for older individuals, namely, determining if the individual is underweight, normal or overweight for height and if the individual is short, medium or tall for his or her age.

Some determination of whether newborn infants are obese, normal or lean can and should be made by inspection and palpation. Determinations of different degrees of obesity and thinness can be made by calculating weight-height ratios or ponderal indices or by measuring skin-fold thickness at appropriate sites. We have used a ponderal index based on Rohrer's formula as follows: birth weight in gm ÷ (crown-heel length in cm³) × 100; this formula was derived from the observation that the weight of an object of uniform density and dimensions increases as the cube of its length.[1] The advantage of the method is that in full-term infants of ≥ 38 weeks or ≥ 48.5 cm in body length, the ponderal index apparently is not affected significantly by race, sex or gestational age.[2, 3] The disadvantage in using this formula is that the error in measuring body length is also cubed. The ponderal index is affected to a definite but slight degree by maternal parity. In brief, some full-term infants born to multiparas are more overweight for their heights than are infants born to primiparas. Clinicians should be prepared to see more obese infants born to multiparas than to primiparas. The explanation for the increased incidence of obesity among later-born infants may relate to the well-recognized increased weight of multiparas in general and possibly to an increased risk of the prediabetic state associated with added years and weight in some multiparas. The ponderal indices of premature infants are significantly affected by gestational age, because soft tissue mass, especially fat, is accumulating more rapidly than growth in body length is occurring. The relative ease with which degrees of obesity and thinness can be determined in newborn infants by using weight-height ratios or ponderal indices has not been generally appreciated by clinicians and investigators, judging by the paucity of these calculations in the literature. Care should be exercised in differentiating between subcutaneous fat and edema in drawing conclusions about the nutritional status and habitus of fetuses and newborn infants.

The matter of determining if fetuses or newborn infants are too large or too small in external body dimensions for their gestational ages is more complicated than estimating degrees of obesity and thinness. However, it is less complicated than determining if birth weight is large, appropriate or small for gestational age. Birth weight is significantly affected by more basic factors than is crown-heel length or head size. Birth weight is affected by the same factors that affect crown-heel length, namely, maternal height, gestational age and infant's sex, and, in addition, birth weight is affected by parity of the mother and her height-weight ratio, neither of which appears to affect crown-heel length significantly. Obviously, the determination of the external dimensions of the fetus in relation to gestational age is of primary importance to the obstetrician and it should be of more concern to the pediatrician than it has been. There is increasing evidence that the length of a baby at birth has predictive value for growth in height—at least during the early postnatal years.[4-6] Sabbagha's study suggests that the size of the infant at birth already may be largely fixed by the twentieth week of pregnancy.[7]

The diagnosis of atypical intrauterine growth depends to a considerable extent on the selection of infants who serve as controls. Previous investigators generally have excluded infants from their control groups who had major congenital malformations or erythroblastosis and infants born to diabetic, hypertensive or preeclamptic mothers. The exclusions have varied from one publication to another and lack uniformity. Furthermore, no attempt has been made to exclude all infants who have had some fetal or maternal condition of a growth-retarding nature. The conditions for which infants have been excluded from previously published studies are shown in Table 4–1. Failure by previous investigators to exclude all infants associated with any intrauterine growth-retarding factor from their published data may reflect the investigators' desires to present data representative of a given population rather than statistics on normally grown fetuses. The problem in excluding all infants with any fetal or maternal growth-retarding condition from tables of standards is the large number of infants who may have to be excluded. This is especially true in tertiary medical centers, which generally have been the sources for supplying data for fetal growth standards. Among infants born at The University of Kansas Medical Center, about 2 of every 3 full-term infants and about 85% of all premature infants have had to be excluded from control groups because of some fetal or maternal growth-retarding factor. Cigarette smoking during pregnancy, which has not been a reason for excluding infants from previously published standards, occurred in 40% of women delivered at The University of Kansas Medical Center during the period of 5 years covered by this study. The Surgeon General of the United States estimated that, on the average, infants of mothers smoking cigarettes during pregnancy weighed 180 gm less at birth than infants of nonsmoking mothers.[17] The data presented in the accompanying tables were obtained on infants who had none of the fetal or maternal growth-retarding conditions listed in Table 3–1 and none of whose mothers had gestational diabetes or diabetes mellitus. Data on premature infants (< 37 completed weeks of gestation) are presented separately from data on full-term infants because there were too few premature infants available for statistical analysis who were not involved with some growth-retarding condition.

Infants were included in the accompanying tables and graphs on standards only if their gestational ages were known and their calculated and estimated gestational ages were in agreement. Gestational age was calculated in completed weeks from the first

TABLE 4-1.—DATA ON PREVIOUSLY PUBLISHED
STANDARDS OF FETAL GROWTH

AUTHORS AND REFERENCE NUMBERS	YEAR PUBLISHED	PARAMETERS MEASURED	EXCLUSIONS	INCLUSIONS
Lubchenco, Hansman and Boyd[8]	1966	Birth weight, length and head circumference	Non-whites, gross malformations, Rh disease, diabetes	Admissions to Colorado General Hospital, 1948-1961
Gruenwald[9]	1966	Birth weight	Multiple births	Births at Sinai Hospital, Baltimore
Hendricks[10]	1964	Birth weight	Multiple births, stillbirths, preeclamptics, diabetics	Births at University Hospitals of Cleveland, 1956-1962
Usher and McLean[11]	1969	Birth weight, length and head circumference	Multiple births, congenital malformations, diabetics	300 births in Montreal, 1959
Babson[12]	1970	Birth weight, length and head circumference	—	Used Usher and McLean's data
Thompson, Billewicz and Hytten[13]	1970	Birth weight	Multiple births, congenital malformations, macerated stillborn and in some tables also preeclamptics and hypertensives	Nearly all births in Aberdeen, Scotland, 1948-1964
Tanner and Thomson[14]	1970	Birth weight	See reference 11	See reference 11
Babson and Benda[15]	1976	Birth weight, length and head circumference	—	Other North American standards
Hoffman, Stark, Lundin and Ashbrook[16]	1974	Birth weight	Multiple births	Births and fetal deaths in 36 states and District of Columbia, 1968

day of the mother's last menstrual period. Gestational age was
estimated by obstetricians relying on pelvic examinations done
early in the first trimester, ultrasonic measurements of biparietal
diameters between 20 and 28 weeks of pregnancy and time of
appearance of fetal heart sounds. After birth, use was made of the
criteria proposed by Dubowitz *et al.*[18] to estimate gestational age.
The infants were born consecutively at The University of Kansas
Medical Center. There were more than 1200 white infants included in the tables on standards and they were about equally
divided between boys and girls and between primiparas and
multiparas. Body measurements were all made by one person
(HCM) and almost always within 48 hours of the infants' births,
using the method described in Chapter 1. Birth weights were
obtained on admission to the newborn nurseries by a previously
described technique.[2] No full-term infants dying in the perinatal
period were included. The data on body lengths, head sizes and
birth weights were grouped according to percentiles at succes-
sive weeks of gestation and the percentile lines smoothed visual-
ly. Data in the tables represent points on the percentile lines after smoothing. The tables on standards are grouped at the end of
this chapter (Tables 4-2, 4-3, 4-7, 4-8, 4-10, 4-11, 4-12 and
4-13).

Crown-heel length. — The distribution of crown-heel lengths
of more than 1200 control infants is shown for full-term boys and
girls according to their gestational ages in Tables 4-2 and 4-3,
respectively. The data in these two tables should not be con-
strued as defining a fetal growth curve for body length. Body
measurements made at one point in time obviously do not, strict-
ly speaking, constitute a growth curve. On the other hand, it is
apparent from the tables that fetal growth in body length is affected by gestational age and sex. Body lengths of newborn infants are also affected by maternal height. Crown-heel lengths of
control boys and girls born to tall mothers not only tended to be
longer than the crown-heel lengths of control boys and girls born
to short mothers (Figs. 4-1 to 4-4) but also more boys and girls
of short mothers tended to have crown-heel lengths that were at
or below the twenty-fifth percentiles for gestational ages. (The
percentile lines in Figs. 4-1 to 4-4 conform to data shown in
Tables 4-2 and 4-3.) However, it was interesting to observe
that short mothers of control infants gave birth to no infants with

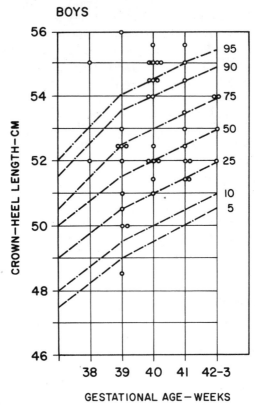

Fig. 4–1.—Crown-heel lengths at birth of boys born to control mothers ≥ 172.9 cm (≥ 68 in.) tall.

crown-heel lengths below the fifth percentiles in Figures 4–1 and 4–2. This observation was quite contrary to the pregnancy outcome for infants of short mothers who had medical complications and behavioral conditions of pregnancy (Chap. 6). The group of infants of short mothers with complications and behavioral conditions of pregnancy as defined in Table 3–1 had a high incidence of boys and girls whose crown-heel lengths at birth were at or below the fifth percentile.

Mean crown-heel lengths of control full-term infants apparently were not affected significantly by parity or by prepregnant

BOYS

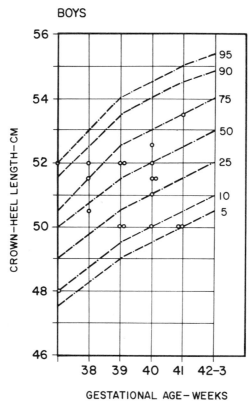

Fig. 4–2. — Crown-heel lengths at birth of boys born to control mothers ≤ 150 cm (≤ 59 in.) tall.

weight-height ratios of mothers (Table 4–4). Twelve groups of infants are shown in Table 4–4; in only 2 of the 12 groups, i.e., later-born boys at 40 weeks and later-born girls at 39 weeks, were there any notable increases in mean body lengths as maternal prepregnancy weight-height ratios increased from ≥ 7.5% below normal to ≥ 7.5% above normal weight for height. The mean crown-heel lengths of later-born infants were not consistently significantly greater than those of first-born infants.

Ponderal index. — The ponderal index is one way of quantifying the degree of obesity and thinness of an infant. Care needs to

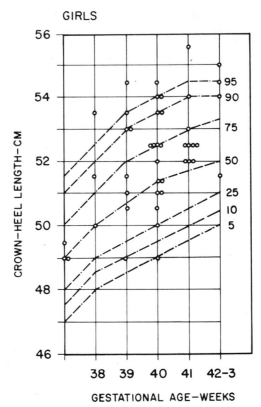

Fig. 4–3. — Crown-heel lengths at birth of girls born to control mothers ≥ 172.9 cm (≥ 68 in.) tall.

be taken in interpreting ponderal indices of infants with disproportionately large or small heads. The head of a fetus or of a newborn infant is such a large part of the body weight that the ponderal index will be distorted if the head is disproportionately large or small, as it occasionally is in a small percentage of fetuses and newborn infants. The percentile distribution of ponderal indices of more than 1200 white control full-term infants in this study is shown in Table 4–5. Comparison of indices of first-born and later-born infants in the table shows that at the ninetieth and ninety-fifth percentiles the ponderal indices of later-born infants

GIRLS

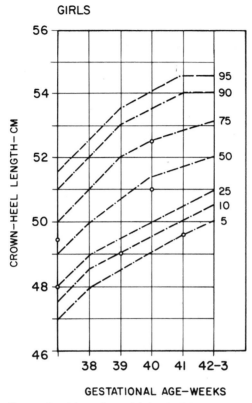

Fig. 4–4. – Crown-heel lengths at birth of girls born to control mothers ≤ 150 cm (≤ 59 in.) tall.

were greater than those of first-born infants, indicating that more infants of multipara were likely to be obese. In clinical practice, we use the distribution of ponderal indices obtained on later-born infants, shown in Table 4–5, to estimate degrees of obesity and thinness on first-born as well as later-born infants. Infants are considered extremely obese who have ponderal indices above 2.93 (95%) and extremely malnourished if their ponderal indices are below 2.26 (5%). Moderate obesity is considered in infants with ponderal indices between 2.85 and 2.93; moderate malnutrition pertains to infants with ponderal indices between 2.32 and 2.26.

TABLE 4–4.—MEAN CROWN-HEEL (C-H) LENGTHS (cm)
AT BIRTH OF WHITE FULL-TERM CONTROL INFANTS
ACCORDING TO PREPREGNANCY HABITUS OF MOTHERS
WHOSE HEIGHTS WERE FROM 157.7 cm (62 in.)
TO 172.9 cm (68 in.)

WEEKS OF GESTATION	MATERNAL[°] WEIGHT-HEIGHT RATIO, PREPREGNANCY	FIRST-BORN		LATER-BORN	
		Boys C-H Length (cm)	Girls C-H Length (cm)	Boys C-H Length (cm)	Girls C-H Length (cm)
39	≥ 7.5% above normal	(14) 51.1	(18) 50.9	(21) 51.0	(27) 51.7
	Average[†]	(24) 52.0	(28) 51.1	(24) 51.9	(19) 51.0
	≥ 7.5% below normal	(6) 51.4	(8) 51.3	(13) 51.4	(13) 50.0
40	≥ 7.5% above normal	(21) 51.9	(18) 51.1	(29) 52.3	(27) 51.4
	Average[†]	(45) 51.8	(36) 51.1	(30) 52.3	(42) 51.4
	≥ 7.5% below normal	(17) 52.0	(16) 51.3	(25) 51.5	(14) 51.4
41	≥ 7.5% above normal	(16) 52.5	(20) 52.0	(14) 52.4	(19) 52.0
	Average[†]	(20) 52.5	(26) 51.4	(23) 52.8	(17) 52.1
	≥ 7.5% below normal	(14) 52.5	(8) 52.0	(17) 52.5	(13) 51.8

( ) indicates number of infants.
[°]Based on Sargent's table for young women.[19]
[†]From 7.5% above to 7.5% below normal in Sargent's table.

TABLE 4–5.—DISTRIBUTION OF
PONDERAL INDICES AMONG
FULL-TERM WHITE
INFANTS (≥ 37 wk)

FIRST BORN	PERCENTILE	LATER BORN
2.83	95	2.93
2.76	90	2.85
2.67	75	2.67
2.54	50	2.54
2.41	25	2.41
2.32	10	2.32
2.26	5	2.26

TABLE 4-6.—BIRTH WEIGHT (kg) BY PERCENTILES, ACCORDING TO CROWN-HEEL LENGTH

PERCENTILES	CROWN-HEEL LENGTH (cm)														
	48.0	48.5	49.0	49.5	50.0	50.5	51.0	51.5	52.0	52.5	53.0	53.5	54.0	54.5	55.0
95	3.16	3.26	3.36	3.47	3.57	3.68	3.79	3.90	4.02	4.13	4.25	4.37	4.50	4.63	4.76
90	3.05	3.15	3.24	3.35	3.45	3.55	3.66	3.77	3.88	3.99	4.11	4.22	4.34	4.47	4.59
75	2.95	3.04	3.14	3.24	3.33	3.43	3.54	3.64	3.75	3.86	3.97	4.09	4.21	4.33	4.45
50	2.81	2.90	2.98	3.08	3.17	3.27	3.37	3.47	3.57	3.67	3.77	3.87	4.00	4.11	4.21
25	2.67	2.75	2.83	2.92	3.01	3.10	3.19	3.29	3.39	3.48	3.58	3.68	3.80	3.91	4.04
10	2.56	2.65	2.73	2.82	2.90	2.99	3.08	3.17	3.26	3.35	3.45	3.55	3.65	3.76	3.86
5	2.45	2.53	2.61	2.69	2.77	2.86	2.94	3.03	3.12	3.21	3.30	3.40	3.50	3.59	3.69

Weight-height ratios.—For those who prefer weight-height ratios to ponderal indices in the evaluation of infants' nutritional state, data on the percentile distribution of birth weights of more than 1200 full-term control infants are shown in Table 4–6 according to their crown-heel lengths at birth. Boys and girls of primiparas and multiparas were combined in Table 4–6. Full-term control infants less than 48 cm long at birth were too few in number to obtain a reasonable percentile distribution of their weight-height ratios. Full-term infants whose weight-height ratios fall below the fifth percentile for their heights should be extremely thin and probably malnourished and should be treated accordingly.

Head size.—The percentile distribution of occipitofrontal (OF) circumferences of more than 1200 full-term control boys and girls is shown in Tables 4–7 and 4–8 according to their gestational ages. Gestational age and sex affected head size. Boys had larger heads than girls. Parity of mothers did not consistently affect head circumferences significantly (Table 4–9). Data in Table 4–9 reveal that in 9 of the 12 groups of infants mean OF circumferences were larger in infants of mothers whose weight-

TABLE 4–9.—MEAN OCCIPITOFRONTAL (OF)
CIRCUMFERENCES (cm) OF FULL-TERM CONTROL
INFANTS ACCORDING TO PREPREGNANCY HABITUS OF
MOTHERS WHOSE HEIGHTS WERE FROM 157.7 cm (62 in.)
TO 172.9 cm (68 in.)

| | | HEAD SIZE | | | |
| | | First-born | | Later-born | |
WEEKS OF GESTATION	MATERNAL° WEIGHT-HEIGHT RATIO, PREPREGNANCY	Boys OF Circ. (cm)	Girls OF Circ. (cm)	Boys OF Circ. (cm)	Girls OF Circ. (cm)
39	≥ 7.5% above normal	(13) 34.6	(20) 34.6	(23) 34.8	(27) 34.7
	Average†	(24) 34.9	(30) 34.3	(21) 34.5	(18) 34.6
	≥ 7.5% below normal	(5) 34.6	(7) 34.0	(10) 34.7	(11) 33.7
40	≥ 7.5% above normal	(23) 35.1	(16) 34.5	(30) 35.7	(29) 34.6
	Average†	(43) 35.0	(38) 35.0	(29) 35.1	(35) 34.5
	≥ 7.5% below normal	(15) 35.0	(16) 34.0	(26) 34.8	(13) 34.0
41	≥ 7.5% above normal	(14) 35.2	(20) 35.1	(16) 35.7	(18) 34.8
	Average†	(20) 35.2	(29) 34.9	(25) 35.7	(16) 34.6
	≥ 7.5% below normal	(15) 35.3	(8) 34.9	(17) 35.0	(13) 34.6

( ) indicates number of infants.
°Based on Sargent's table for young women.[19]
†From 7.5% above to 7.5% below normal in Sargent's table.

height ratios before pregnancy were above average than in infants of mothers whose weight-height ratios were below average. In some of the 9 groups, the mean OF circumferences were from 0.5 to 1.0 cm larger. The effect of maternal height on OF circumferences of full-term control infants was much less than the effect of maternal height on crown-heel lengths. Head circumferences of consecutively born control infants of tall mothers are shown in Figure 4–5 and of short mothers in Figure 4–6. The mothers of infants whose head sizes are plotted in Figures 4–5 and 4–6 were all of average prepregnancy body weight for height. There appears to be little difference between the head circumferences of these two groups of infants, as plotted in Figures 4–5 and 4–6.

Birth weight. — Birth weights were affected by gestational age and sex of infant and maternal height, parity and prepregnancy weight-height ratio. Boys were heavier than girls and later-born infants were heavier than first-born infants, as shown in Tables

Fig. 4–5. — Head circumferences of boys (●) and girls (○) at birth born to control mothers of average weight for height and ≥ 172.9 cm (≥ 68 in.) tall.

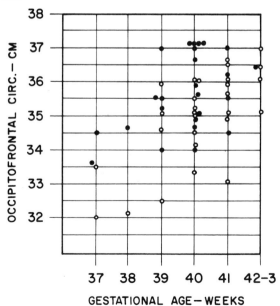

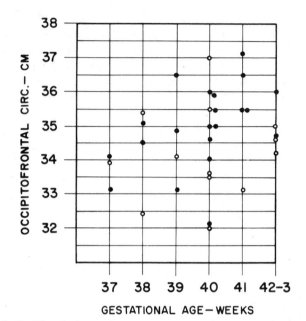

GESTATIONAL AGE — WEEKS

Fig. 4–6.—Head circumferences of boys (●) and girls (○) at birth born to control mothers of average weight for height and ≤ 152.6 cm (≤ 60 in.) tall.

TABLE 4–14.—MEAN BIRTH WEIGHTS (BW) OF WHITE FULL-TERM CONTROL INFANTS ACCORDING TO PREPREGNANCY HABITUS OF MOTHERS WHOSE HEIGHTS WERE FROM 157.7 cm (62 in.) TO 172.9 cm (68 in.)

		FIRST-BORN		LATER-BORN	
WEEKS OF GESTATION	MATERNAL° WEIGHT-HEIGHT RATIO, PREPREGNANCY	Boys BW (kg)	Girls BW (kg)	Boys BW (kg)	Girls BW (kg)
39	≥ 7.5% above normal	(16) 3.48	(21) 3.41	(23) 3.48	(27) 3.58
	Average†	(25) 3.46	(28) 3.41	(25) 3.45	(18) 3.58
	≥ 7.5% below normal	(5) 3.36	(8) 3.36	(10) 3.46	(11) 3.21
40	≥ 7.5% above normal	(22) 3.49	(19) 3.55	(27) 3.71	(31) 3.60
	Average†	(45) 3.50	(36) 3.44	(30) 3.57	(37) 3.45
	≥ 7.5% below normal	(16) 3.43	(14) 3.45	(24) 3.56	(13) 3.44
41	≥ 7.5% above normal	(16) 3.67	(22) 3.61	(15) 3.87	(16) 3.59
	Average†	(17) 3.69	(26) 3.48	(26) 3.81	(17) 3.66
	≥ 7.5% below normal	(14) 3.67	(9) 3.58	(15) 3.53	(14) 3.46

( ) indicates number of infants.
°Based on Sargent's table for young women.[19]
†From 7.5% above to 7.5% below normal in Sargent's table.

4-10 to 4-13. Data in Table 4-14 on 12 groups of infants at three different gestational ages show that mothers of average height who were overweight for their heights at conception consistently (in 11 of 12 groups) had heavier babies than did mothers who were underweight; in the twelfth group, the mean birth weights were not significantly different between infants of overweight and underweight mothers. When prepregnancy habitus of control mothers was controlled by removing all overweight and underweight mothers and by taking only mothers with average weight-height ratios, it was observed that tall mothers had heavier babies than did short mothers, as shown in Figures 4-7 to 4-10. The effect of maternal height on the birth weight of infants was almost certainly dependent on the effect of maternal height on body lengths of fetuses.

Fig. 4-7.—Birth weights of first-born boys (●) and later-born boys (x) born to control mothers of average weight for height and ≥ 172.9 cm (≥ 68 in.) tall.

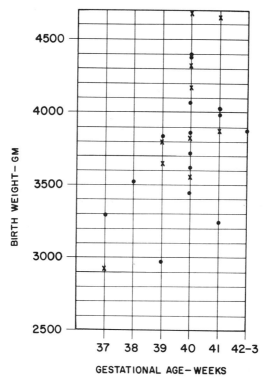

BIRTH WEIGHT — GM

GESTATIONAL AGE — WEEKS

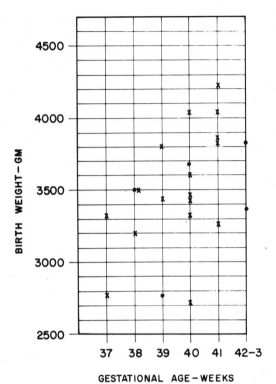

Fig. 4—8. — Birth weights of first-born boys (●) and of later-born boys (x) born to control mothers of average weight for height and ≤ 152.6 cm (≤ 60 in.) tall.

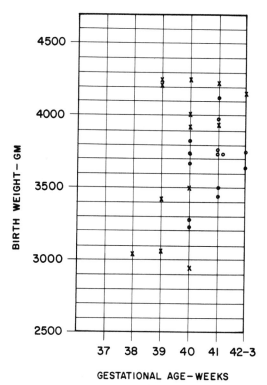

Fig. 4-9.—Birth weights of first-born girls (●) and of later-born girls (x) born to control mothers of average weight for height and ≧ 172.9 cm (≧ 68 in.) tall.

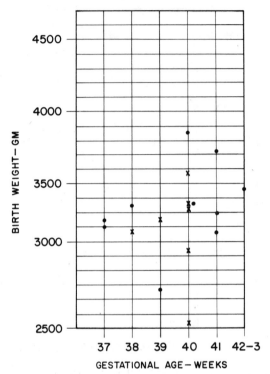

Fig. 4–10.—Birth weights of first-born girls (●) and of later-born girls (x) born to control mothers of average weight for height and ≤ 152.6 cm (≤ 60 in.) tall.

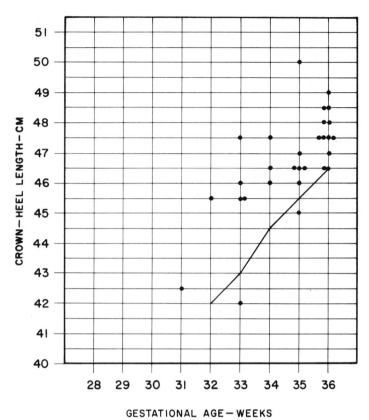

Fig. 4–11. — Crown-heel lengths at birth of premature infants born to control mothers. Solid line is median of crown-heel lengths of premature infants born to mothers with fetal growth-retarding factors.

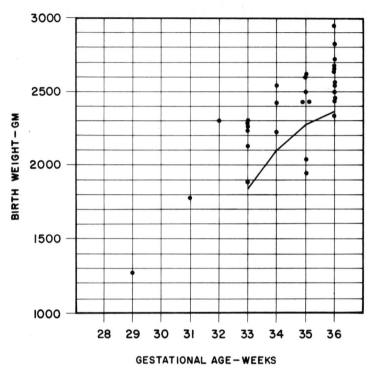

Fig. 4–12. — Birth weights of premature infants born to control mothers. Solid line is median of birth weights of premature infants born to mothers with fetal growth-retarding factors.

Premature infants. — It was not possible to construct the usual types of fetal growth curves based on premature infants born to control white mothers at The University of Kansas Medical Center because there were too few of them. Less than 20% of all white premature infants born at this university could be classified as controls, i.e., born to mothers with no known growth-retarding factors in their pregnancies. The few control premature infants (< 37 completed weeks of gestation) generally were at the more advanced gestational ages and all but 3 of the 30 controls had birth weights over 2000 gm. The birth lengths and weights of the control group are plotted in Figures 4–11 and 4–12, respectively; birth lengths and weights of study premature infants born to mothers with medical complications of pregnancy or

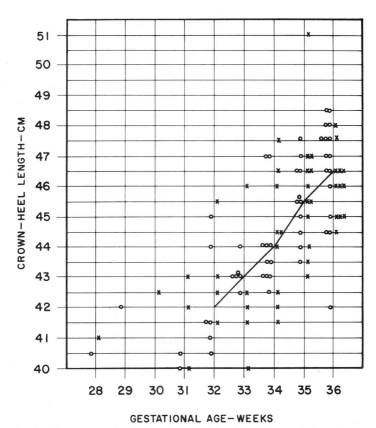

Fig. 4–13. — Crown-heel lengths at birth of premature infants born to mothers with medical complications of pregnancy (x) or with behavioral conditions of pregnancy (O). Solid line is median of their birth weights.

with behavioral conditions listed in Table 3–1 are plotted in Figures 4–13 and 4–14, respectively. Using the student's t test, the crown-heel lengths of control premature infants at 33, 34, 35 and 36 weeks of gestation were significantly longer than those of study infants at similar ages, the p values being 0.014, 0.0017, 0.045 and 0.004, respectively. The birth weights of control infants born at 33 and 36 weeks were significantly greater than those of study infants at similar weeks of gestation, the p values being 0.003 and 0.00009, respectively. In each of the figures, the

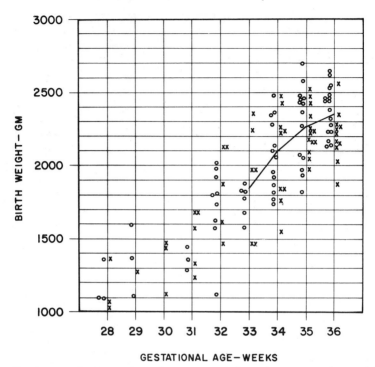

Fig. 4–14.—Birth weights of premature infants born to mothers with medical complications of pregnancy (x) or with behavioral conditions of pregnancy (O). Solid line is median of their birth weights.

solid line represents the median crown-heel lengths or median birth weights of premature infants in the respective study groups.

One would expect that premature infants who were born to control mothers would have a better prognosis for immediate and long-range survival and development than premature infants in the study groups, who were generally less mature and some of whom probably were growth retarded. Until intrauterine growth curves for premature infants can be based on infants born to women free from medical complications and other growth-retarding factors, it would seem highly desirable to signify whether or not premature infants were born to mothers with potential growth-retarding factors in their pregnancies and not to treat all premature infants as though they had been normally grown in utero.

TABLE 4-2.—DISTRIBUTION OF CROWN-HEEL
LENGTHS (cm) OF WHITE NEWBORN MALE
INFANTS (controls) BY PERCENTILES
ACCORDING TO THEIR GESTATIONAL AGES

PERCENTILES	GESTATIONAL AGE—WEEKS					
	37	38	39	40	41	42-43
95	52.0	53.0	54.0	54.5	55.0	55.3
90	51.5	52.5	53.5	54.0	54.5	54.8
75	50.5	51.5	52.5	53.0	53.5	54.0
50	50.0	50.7	51.5	52.0	52.5	53.0
25	49.0	49.7	50.5	51.0	51.5	52.0
10	48.0	48.7	49.5	50.0	50.5	51.0
5	47.5	48.2	49.0	49.5	50.0	50.5

TABLE 4-3.—DISTRIBUTION OF CROWN-HEEL (cm)
LENGTHS OF WHITE NEWBORN FEMALE
INFANTS (controls) BY PERCENTILES
ACCORDING TO THEIR GESTATIONAL AGES

PERCENTILES	GESTATIONAL AGE—WEEKS					
	37	38	39	40	41	42-43
95	51.5	52.5	53.5	54.0	54.5	54.5
90	51.0	52.0	53.0	53.5	54.0	54.0
75	50.0	51.0	52.0	52.5	52.8	53.1
50	49.0	50.0	50.7	51.3	51.7	52.0
25	48.0	48.9	49.5	50.0	50.5	51.0
10	47.5	48.5	49.0	49.5	50.0	50.5
5	47.0	47.9	48.6	49.1	49.5	50.0

TABLE 4-7.—DISTRIBUTION OF OCCIPITOFRONTAL
CIRCUMFERENCES (cm) OF WHITE NEWBORN
MALE INFANTS (controls) BY PERCENTILES
ACCORDING TO THEIR GESTATIONAL AGES

PERCENTILES	GESTATIONAL AGE—WEEKS					
	37	38	39	40	41	42-43
95	35.5	36.0	36.4	36.8	37.2	37.4
90	35.2	35.6	35.9	36.3	36.7	37.2
75	34.6	34.9	35.3	35.7	36.0	36.2
50	34.0	34.3	34.6	34.9	35.2	35.5
25	33.4	33.7	34.0	34.3	34.7	35.0
10	32.8	33.2	33.5	33.8	34.2	34.5
5	32.4	32.7	33.1	33.4	33.8	34.2

TABLE 4-8.—DISTRIBUTION OF OCCIPITOFRONTAL
CIRCUMFERENCES (cm) OF WHITE NEWBORN
FEMALE INFANTS (controls) BY PERCENTILES
ACCORDING TO THEIR GESTATIONAL AGES

	GESTATIONAL AGE — WEEKS					
PERCENTILES	37	38	39	40	41	42-43
95	35.0	35.5	35.9	36.2	36.5	36.8
90	34.5	35.0	35.4	35.7	36.1	36.3
75	33.9	34.3	34.7	35.1	35.5	35.8
50	33.2	33.6	34.1	34.5	34.8	35.2
25	32.5	32.9	33.4	33.8	34.2	34.5
10	32.0	32.4	32.8	33.2	33.6	33.9
5	31.8	32.2	32.6	32.9	33.3	33.6

TABLE 4-10.—PERCENTILE DISTRIBUTION OF
BIRTH WEIGHTS (kg) OF WHITE FIRST-BORN
MALE INFANTS (controls) ACCORDING TO
THEIR GESTATIONAL AGES

	GESTATIONAL AGE — WEEKS					
PERCENTILES	37	38	39	40	41	42-43
95	3.63	3.82	3.97	4.10	4.23	4.34
90	3.50	3.70	3.86	4.00	4.13	4.24
75	3.30	3.48	3.65	3.78	3.92	4.03
50	3.10	3.27	3.43	3.57	3.70	3.82
25	2.85	3.00	3.13	3.26	3.38	3.49
10	2.70	2.84	2.96	3.08	3.18	3.28
5	2.62	2.76	2.88	3.00	3.10	3.20

TABLE 4-11.—PERCENTILE DISTRIBUTION OF
BIRTH WEIGHTS (kg) OF WHITE FIRST-BORN
FEMALE INFANTS (controls) ACCORDING TO
THEIR GESTATIONAL AGES

	GESTATIONAL AGE — WEEKS					
PERCENTILES	37	38	39	40	41	42-43
95	3.44	3.72	3.90	4.03	4.12	4.20
90	3.30	3.60	3.80	3.92	4.02	4.10
75	3.17	3.38	3.57	3.70	3.82	3.94
50	3.00	3.15	3.30	3.43	3.56	3.66
25	2.79	2.93	3.07	3.18	3.29	3.37
10	2.55	2.72	2.85	2.97	3.09	3.17
5	2.46	2.61	2.76	2.89	3.01	3.10

TABLE 4-12.—PERCENTILE DISTRIBUTION OF
BIRTH WEIGHTS (kg) OF WHITE MALE
INFANTS (controls) BORN TO MULTIPARAS
ACCORDING TO INFANTS' GESTATIONAL AGES

PERCENTILES	GESTATIONAL AGE—WEEKS					
	37	38	39	40	41	42-43
95	3.66	4.00	4.20	4.39	4.50	4.60
90	3.47	3.70	3.90	4.08	4.24	4.37
75	3.30	3.50	3.70	3.87	4.03	4.15
50	3.10	3.27	3.44	3.61	3.75	3.85
25	2.85	3.02	3.18	3.34	3.50	3.62
10	2.71	2.86	3.02	3.19	3.34	3.45
5	2.63	2.78	2.94	3.08	3.21	3.32

TABLE 4-13.—PERCENTILE DISTRIBUTION OF
BIRTH WEIGHTS (kg) OF WHITE FEMALE
INFANTS (controls) BORN TO MULTIPARAS
ACCORDING TO INFANTS' GESTATIONAL AGES

PERCENTILES	GESTATIONAL AGE—WEEKS					
	37	38	39	40	41	42-43
95	3.60	3.86	4.02	4.14	4.23	4.31
90	3.50	3.67	3.84	3.95	4.07	4.15
75	3.26	3.48	3.64	3.75	3.85	3.95
50	3.00	3.20	3.34	3.50	3.62	3.72
25	2.80	2.95	3.08	3.23	3.35	3.45
10	2.67	2.80	2.93	3.05	3.16	3.26
5	2.52	2.67	2.80	2.92	3.04	3.15

REFERENCES

1. Rohrer, F.: Der Index der Körperfülle als Mass des Ern-
ährungszustandes, Münch. Med. Wochenschr. 68:580, 1921.
2. Miller, H. C., and Hassanein, K.: Diagnosis of impaired fetal growth
in newborn infants, Pediatrics 48:511, 1971.
3. Miller, H. C.: Fetal growth and neonatal mortality, Pediatrics 49:
392, 1972.
4. Garn, S. M., Shaw, H. A., and McCabe, K. D.: Birth size and growth
appraisal, J. Pediatr. 90:1049, 1977.
5. Smith, D. W., Truog, W., Rogers, J. E., Greitzer, L. J., Skinner, A. L.,
McCann, J. J., and Harvey, M. A. S.: Shifting linear growth during
infancy. Illustration of genetic factors in growth from fetal life
through infancy, J. Pediatr. 89:225, 1976.
6. Holmes, G. E., Miller, H. C., Hassanein, K., Lansky, S. B., and Goggin, J. E.: Postnatal somatic growth in babies with atypical fetal
growth patterns, Am. J. Dis. Child. 131:1078, 1977.

7. Sabbagha, R. E.: Biparietal diameter: An appraisal, Clini. Obstet. Gynaecol. 21:297, 1977.

8. Lubchenco, L. O., Hansman, C., and Boyd, E.: Intrauterine growth in length and head circumference as estimated from live births at gestational ages from 26 to 42 weeks, Pediatrics 37:403, 1966.

9. Gruenwald, P.: Growth of the human fetus. 1. Normal growth and its variation, Am. J. Obstet. Gynecol. 94:1112, 1966.

10. Hendricks, C. H.: Patterns of fetal and placental growth: The second half of normal pregnancy, Obstet. Gynecol. 24:357, 1964.

11. Usher, R., and McLean, F.: Intrauterine growth of live-bron Caucasian infants at sea level: Standards obtained from measurements in 7 dimensions of infants born between 25 and 44 weeks of gestation, J. Pediatr. 74:901, 1969.

12. Babson, S. G.: Growth of low-birth-weight infants, J. Pediatr. 77:11, 1970.

13. Thomson, A. M., Billewicz, W. Z., and Hytten, F. E.: The assessment of fetal growth, J. Obstet. Gynaecol. Br. Commonw. 75:903, 1970.

14. Tanner, J. M., and Thomson, A. M.: Standards for birth weight at gestation periods from 32 to 42 weeks, allowing for maternal height and weight, Arch. Dis. Child. 45:506, 1970.

15. Babson, S. G., and Benda, G. I.: Growth graphs for the clinical assessment of infants of varying gestational ages, J. Pediatr. 89:814, 1976.

16. Hoffman, H. J., Stark, C. R., Lundin, F. E., and Ashbrook, J. D.: Analysis of birth weight, gestational age and fetal viability, U. S. births, 1968, Obstet. Gynecol. Surv. 29:651, 1974.

17. United States Public Health Service: The health consequences of smoking: Reports of the Surgeon General (Washington, D. C.: Government Printing Office, 1971, 1972, 1973).

18. Dubowitz, L. M. S., Dubowitz, V., and Goldberg, C.: Clinical assessment of gestational age in the newborn infant, J. Pediatr. 77:1, 1970.

19. Sargent, D. W.: Weight-height relationship of young men and women, J. Nutr. 13:318, 1963.

5 / Socioeconomic Factors

MANY REPORTS over the years from around the world fully support the observation that infants born to mothers in low socioeconomic circumstances weigh less at birth than infants born under better circumstances.[1-7] Efforts made to identify specific social and economic factors to account for these lower birth weights have been singularly unrewarding. Naylor and Myrianthopoulos[8] investigated the effects of eleven different social and economic factors on the birth weights of infants in the Collaborative Study on Cerebral Palsy carried out under the aegis of the National Institutes of Health. The eleven factors included place of birth (urban or rural, within and outside the continental United States), education of gravida, occupation of gravida, religion, marital status, housing density, presence or absence of father in home, education of husband, occupation of husband, family income and income from welfare sources. They concluded, "While the regression of birth weight on many socio-economic variables is highly significant, very little of the variance in birth weight is accounted for by these variables." Morris and associates[9] concluded from a study of unwanted pregnancies that "prevention of the unwanted pregnancies will cause no practical reduction in overall low birth weight (< 2500 gm) birth rates." Rosen and his group[4] observed that illegitimacy among mothers delivered at Harlem Hospital in New York City was not associated with a greater number of low-weight babies. Studies previously reported from The University of Kansas Medical Center suggested that social and economic factors were not primarily responsible for the increased births of low birth weight (LBW) infants among women of poor socioeconomic status, but rather the increase in LBW infants appeared to be dependent on choices that mothers made with respect to their pregnancies, such as cigarette smoking and the other behavioral conditions listed in Table 3–1.[10, 11] The adoption by mothers of the seven

behavioral conditions listed in Table 3–1 increased the risk of
fetal growth retardation and of premature births (< 37 weeks),
irrespective of maternal socioeconomic circumstances. The important fact was that women in the lowest socioeconomic group
were far more likely to adopt one or more of the seven behavioral
conditions listed in Table 3–1 than were women in the highest
socioeconomic group. For example, the incidence of women
smoking cigarettes during pregnancy was 60% in the lowest and
15% in the highest socioeconomic group and low weight gains in
pregnancy were 3 times more likely to occur among women in
the lowest than in the highest socioeconomic group. The incidence of chronic alcoholism and drug addiction was inverse to
socioeconomic status.

In this chapter, we have expanded the number of women and
their infants previously reported from The University of Kansas
Medical Center.[10, 11] A low birth weight (< 2500 gm) was used as
the criterion in evaluating the effects of socioeconomic factors
on fetal outcome for the reason that all pregnancies can be
included. If either mean birth weight or mean crown-heel length
had been used as criteria, pregnancies in which gestational age
was unknown or uncertain would have needed to be excluded
and there would have been more exclusions in the lower than
in the higher socioeconomic groups, because women in the
lower groups tended to be less certain of their pregnancy dates
than women in the higher socioeconomic groups. By making
LBW infants the dependent variable there is need only to
distinguish between premature and full-term infants, and even
that distinction can be waived.

Data in the accompanying tables include more than 2700
white mothers and their single infants. The mothers were
delivered consecutively at The University of Kansas Medical
Center and were part of the prospective study on fetal growth
that began here in 1973. Taylor's job classification was used in
determining the occupations of heads of households.[12] All
mothers were classified by the Admitting Office of the Medical
Center as belonging to either the nonpoverty or the poverty
group. The poverty group conformed to guidelines established
in 1974 by the United States Department of Labor.[13] Mothers in
the nonpoverty group were charged full hospital costs and a
physician's fee. Mothers in the poverty group were either

unemployed, on welfare or had their hospital expenses discounted; physicians' fees included only the amounts allowed by third-party payments. Class I in the nonpoverty group included persons in professional or managerial positions. Class II in the nonpoverty group included manual, clerical, service and sales personnel. Class III in the poverty group included the same personnel as in Class II. Class IV in the poverty group were unemployed and most were on welfare. The diagnosis of maternal complications of pregnancy was taken from the obstetric records of the mothers by one of us (HCM), who also interviewed each mother and measured and evaluated each infant as set forth in a previous publication.[14]

Mothers and infants were divided into three groups. One group included mothers with medical complications of pregnancy as listed in Table 3–1; another group had one or more of the seven behavioral conditions listed in the same table, but none of the medical complications of pregnancy in Table 3–1 and the third group served as a control group and had none of the factors listed in Table 3–1. All infants with fetal conditions as listed in Table 3–1 were excluded from Table 5–1. The total incidence of LBW infants in each of the three groups is shown in Table 5–1 and ranged from 1.7% in the control group to 9.8% in the group

TABLE 5–1.–INCIDENCE OF LOW BIRTH WEIGHT
INFANTS (< 2500 gm) ACCORDING TO THE PRESENCE
AND ABSENCE OF FETAL GROWTH-RETARDING
FACTORS IN GRAVIDAS

NO. OF GRAVIDAS WITH FETAL GROWTH-RETARDING FACTORS	LOW BIRTH WEIGHT (LBW) INFANTS					
	Premature (< 37 Weeks)		Full-term (≥ 37 Weeks)		Total LBW Infants	
	No.	%	No.	%	No.	%
No growth-retarding factors (1088)	11	1.0	7	0.6	18	1.7
Behavioral* conditions (1269)	88	6.9	36	2.8	124	9.8
Medical complications† of pregnancy (429)	64	14.9	24	5.6	88	20.5
Total gravidas (2786)	163	5.9	67	2.4	230	8.2

*Behavioral conditions: (1) cigarette smoking, (2) addicting drugs or chronic alcoholism, (3) underweight at conception, (4) low maternal weight gain, (5) no prenatal care, delivery before (6) seventeenth or after (7) thirty-fifth birthdays.
†Medical complications, as listed under group II, Table 3–1.

with behavioral conditions and 20.5% in the group with medical complications of pregnancy. The data in Table 5–1 show that the incidence of LBW premature and full-term infants was low in the control group of mothers, was higher among mothers with behavioral conditions and was highest in the group of mothers with medical complications. The differences are significant, $p < 0.05$, by the Z test, taking the multiple comparisons into consideration to adjust p. The ratio of premature to full-term infants in the total group of 230 LBW infants was 70 to 30.

In Table 5–2, data show that the incidence of LBW infants born to control mothers was low in all four socioeconomic groups and not significantly different. There were no significant differences in the incidences of LBW infants in the four socioeconomic groups of mothers with behavioral conditions or in the four socioeconomic groups of mothers with medical complications.

The important point to be observed is the distribution of mothers in the four socioeconomic groups (Table 5–3). The incidence of mothers with medical complications was not significantly different in the four socioeconomic groups, but there were significant differences in the incidences of control mothers and mothers with behavioral conditions in the four socioeconomic groups. The group of mothers having the highest socioeconomic status, group I, contained the greatest incidence of control mothers,

TABLE 5–2.–INCIDENCE OF LOW BIRTH WEIGHT (LBW)
INFANTS (< 2500 gm) ACCORDING TO MATERNAL
SOCIOECONOMIC STATUS AND TO PRESENCE AND ABSENCE
OF FETAL GROWTH-RETARDING (G-R) FACTORS IN GRAVIDAS

SOCIOECONOMIC GROUPS	NO G-R FACTORS (controls)			BEHAVIORAL[*] CONDITIONS			MEDICAL[†] COMPLICATIONS		
	Gravidas No.	LBW Infants No.	%	Gravidas No.	LBW Infants No.	%	Gravidas No.	LBW Infants No.	%
Group I	413	7	1.7	193	22	11.4	97	23	23.6
Group II	313	7	2.2	402	37	9.2	155	37	23.9
Group III	167	2	1.2	273	20	7.3	74	11	14.9
Group IV	195	2	1.0	401	45	11.2	103	17	14.7
Total	1088	18	1.7	1269	124	9.8	429	88	20.5

[*]Behavioral conditions same as in Table 5–1.
[†]Medical complications as listed in group II, Table 3–1.

TABLE 5–3.–DISTRIBUTION OF GRAVIDAS IN FOUR
SOCIOECONOMIC GROUPS ACCORDING TO PRESENCE
AND ABSENCE OF FETAL GROWTH-RETARDING (G-R)
FACTORS IN THEIR PREGNANCIES

SOCIOECONOMIC GROUPS	NO. OF GRAVIDAS WITH AND WITHOUT G-R FACTORS							
	No G-R Factors		Behavioral° Conditions		Medical† Complications		TOTAL GRAVIDAS	
	No.	%	No.	%	No.	%	No.	%
Group I	413	58.8	193	27.4	97	13.8	703	100.0
Group II	313	36.0	402	46.2	155	17.8	870	100.0
Group III	167	32.5	273	53.1	74	14.4	514	100.0
Group IV	195	27.9	401	57.4	103	14.7	699	100.0

°Behavioral conditions same as in Table 5–1.
†Medical complications as listed in group II, Table 3–1.

58.8%. The lowest incidence of control mothers, 27.9%, was in
the lowest socioeconomic group, group IV. The difference is significant by the Z test, p < 0.01. The incidence of mothers with
behavioral conditions became progressively larger as socioeconomic status declined; in group I, the incidence was 27.4%
and in group IV it was 57.4%. The difference is significant by the
Z test, p < 0.01. More than half (124) of the total group of 230
LBW infants in this study were born to women with behavioral
conditions in their pregnancies. The unequal distribution of
these women in the four socioeconomic groups consequently
had an important bearing on pregnancy outcome.

It was interesting to observe that control mothers in the lowest
socioeconomic group (group IV) had as little risk of having LBW
infants as mothers in group I and that mothers with behavioral
conditions in group I had the same high risk of having LBW infants as mothers in group IV. If specific socioeconomic factors
were primarily responsible for pregnancy outcome, one would
expect to have observed differences in the incidences of LBW
infants born to control mothers in groups I and IV. The equally
low incidences of LBW infants born to control mothers in groups
I and IV occurred in the presence of marked differences in ages,
educational levels and marital status of the mothers as well as the
already-stated differences in occupations of the head of the
household and in family affluence. More than 95% of mothers in

62 SOCIOECONOMIC FACTORS

socioeconomic group I were married, which was almost twice the rate of married women in group IV. Almost all mothers in group I had some college education and more than half of them had been graduated from college. In group IV, an occasional mother attended college, but less than half of the mothers finished high school and some went only as far as the eighth grade.

The ratio of LBW infants who were premature and full-term in this study compares well with ratios published by other investigators. The group of 67 undergrown full-term LBW infants in Table 5–1 was composed of infants with both types of fetal growth retardation. There were 15 infants who had low ponderal indices (<fifth percentile, Table 4–5); 39 infants were short-for-dates (≤fifth percentiles for their gestation ages, Tables 4–2 and 4–3); 9 infants had both types of fetal growth retardation, i.e., they were both short and lean; 4 full-term infants were not measured but had birth weights under 2500 gm. The ratio of boys to girls in the group of 163 premature LBW infants was 70 to 90; in the group of full-term LBW infants the ratio of boys to girls was 25 to 40.

REFERENCES

1. Abramowicz, M., and Kass, E. H.: Pathogenesis and prognosis of prematurity, N. Engl. J. Med. 275:878, 938, 1001 and 1053, 1966.
2. Bergner, L., and Susser, M. W.: Low birth weight and prenatal nutrition: An interpretative review, Pediatrics 46:946, 1970.
3. Baird, D.: Environmental and obstetrical factors in prematurity with special reference to experience in Aberdeen, Bull. WHO 26:291, 1962.
4. Rosen, M., Downs, E., Napolitani, F. D., and Swartz, D. P.: The quality of reproduction in an urban indigent population, Obstet. Gynecol. 31:276, 1968.
5. Papaevangelou, G., Papadatos, C., and Alexiou, D.: The effect of maternal age, parity and social class on the incidence of small-for-dates newborns, Acta Paediatr. Scand. 62:527, 1973.
6. Hendricks, C. H.: Delivery patterns and reproductive efficiency among groups of differing socioeconomic status and ethnic origins, Am. J. Obstet. Gynecol. 97:608, 1967.
7. Lewis, R., Charles, M., and Patwary, K. M.: Relationships between birth weight and selected social, environmental and medical care factors, Am. J. Public Health 63:973, 1973.
8. Naylor, A. F., and Myrianthopoulos, N. C.: The relation of ethnic and selected socio-economic factors to human birth weight, Ann. Hum. Genet. 31:71, 1967.
9. Morris, N. M., Udry, J. R., and Chase, C. L.: Reduction of low birth

weight birth rates by the prevention of unwanted pregnancies, Am. J. Public Health 63:935, 1973.

10. Miller, H. C., Hassanein, K., Chin, T. D. Y., and Hensleigh, P.: Socioeconomic factors in relation to fetal growth in white infants, J. Pediatr. 89:638, 1976.

11. Miller, H. C., Hassanein, K., and Hensleigh, P.: Effects of behavioral and medical variables on fetal growth retardation, Am. J. Obstet. Gynecol. 127:643, 1977.

12. Taylor, L.: *Occupational Sociology* (New York: Oxford University Press, 1968).

13. U. S. Department of Labor, Manpower Administration, Washington, D. C., News release No. 74-293, June 9, 1974.

14. Miller, H. C., and Hassanein, K.: Diagnosis of impaired fetal growth in newborn infants, Pediatrics 48:511, 1971.

6 / Short and Tall Mothers

THE OPINION is widely held that short women tend to produce smaller newborn infants than do tall women. Belief in this opinion has been supported by studies of other mammals, showing that maternal and not paternal size determines to a large extent the size of the fetus. The Ounsteds[1] have summarized some of these animal studies in their book on fetal growth. The important question in humans that has not been answered is the extent to which maternal stature contributes to the skeletal size of the fetus. In previous studies of this question, maternal stature has not been carefully isolated from the many other factors that are believed capable of inhibiting linear skeletal growth in utero. An additional problem in previous studies has been the heavy reliance on birth weight as the sole determinant of fetal size. There is a correlation between body weight and body size, but body weight is not as ideal or as valid an indicator of size as are external body dimensions. In the Collaborative Perinatal Study of the National Institute of Neurological Diseases and Stroke, an association between the maternal heights of both black and white women and the mean birth weights of their infants was observed.[2] Also, the incidence of low birth weight infants (<2500 gm) was higher among short women than among taller women. Data are presented in this chapter on the association between maternal heights of white mothers delivered consecutively at the University of Kansas Medical Center and the crown-heel lengths and head circumferences of their newborn infants. The effect of maternal height on fetal size was studied by comparing pregnancy outcome in a group of mothers who had none of the growth-retarding factors listed in Table 3–1 in their pregnancies with pregnancy outcome in women who had one or more of the seven behavioral conditions listed in Table 3–1 but none of the other factors listed in that table. None of the mothers in either group had diabetes. The number of mothers in each of the two groups

TABLE 6-1.—DISTRIBUTION OF FULL-TERM CONTROL INFANTS ACCORDING TO THEIR CROWN-HEEL LENGTHS AND TO MATERNAL HEIGHTS

| MATERNAL HEIGHT | | Total infants | CROWN-HEEL LENGTHS (CM) OF FULL-TERM INFANTS | | | | | | MEAN FETAL AGE (WKS) |
| | | | ≥ 51.0 | | 50.5 – 49.0 | | < 49.0 | | |
Cm	In.	No.	No.	%	No.	%	No.	%	
≥170.4	(≥67)	196	167	85.2	26	13.3	3	1.5	40.0
165.3 – 170.3	(65 – 66.9)	195	149	76.4	38	19.5	8	4.1	40.0
160.2 – 165.2	(63 – 64.9)	195	130	66.7	52	26.6	13	6.7	40.0
155.1 – 160.1	(61 – 62.9)	187	104	55.6	62	33.2	21	11.2	39.7
<155.1	(<61)	95	53	55.8	33	34.7	9	9.5	39.8
Total		868	603	69.5	211	24.3	54	6.2	

TABLE 6-2.—DISTRIBUTION OF FULL-TERM INFANTS BORN TO MOTHERS WITH BEHAVIORAL CONDITIONS* ACCORDING TO INFANTS' CROWN-HEEL LENGTHS AND TO MATERNAL HEIGHTS

MATERNAL HEIGHT		CROWN-HEEL LENGTHS (CM) OF FULL-TERM INFANTS							MEAN FETAL AGE (WKS)
Cm	In.	Total infants No.	≥51.0 No.	%	50.5-49.0 No.	%	<49.0 No.	%	
≥170.4	(≥67)	187	109	58.3	63	33.7	15	8.0	39.8
165.3-170.3	(65-66.9)	180	92	51.2	69	38.2	19	10.5	40.0
160.2-165.2	(63-64.9)	185	92	49.7	61	33.0	32	17.3	39.7
155.1-160.1	(61-62.9)	178	67	37.6	76	42.7	35	19.7	39.9
<155.1	(<61)	106	30	28.3	45	32.5	31	29.2	39.9
Total		836	390	46.5	314	37.6	132	15.9	

*(1) Cigarette smoking, (2) addicting drugs or chronic alcoholism, (3) underweight at conception, (4) low maternal weight gain, (5) no prenatal care, (6) delivery before seventeenth or after (7) thirty-fifth birthdays. Mothers with behavioral conditions had none of the other growth-retarding factors in their pregnancies listed in Table 3-1.

was approximately the same. The total number of short mothers under 160.2 cm (63 in.) in height was fewer than the number of tall mothers.

The effect of the heights of 868 control mothers on the crown-heel lengths of their full-term infants is shown in Table 6-1.

TABLE 6-3.—DISTRIBUTION OF FULL-TERM CONTROL INFANTS ACCORDING TO THEIR OCCIPITOFRONTAL CIRCUMFERENCES AND TO THEIR MOTHERS' HEIGHTS

MATERNAL HEIGHT		Total infants No.	OCCIPITOFRONTAL CIRCUMFERENCES (CM) OF FULL-TERM INFANTS						
			≥ 35		34.9–33.0		< 33		Not measured
Cm	In.		No.	%	No.	%	No.	%	No.
≥170.4	(≥67)	196	109	55.6	85	43.3	2	1.0	0
165.3–170.3	(65–66.9)	195	106	54.4	81	41.5	8	4.1	0
160.2–165.2	(63–64.9)	195	85	43.6	97	49.8	13	6.7	0
155.1–160.1	(61–62.9)	187	77	41.2	95	50.9	15	8.0	2
<155.1	(<61)	95	43	43.2	43	45.2	9	9.5	2
Total		868	420	48.4	401	46.2	47	5.4	2

There was a definite association between maternal height and crown-heel length; 85% of infants born to control mothers ≥170.4 cm (67 in.) tall had crown-heel lengths of 51 cm or more, but only 55% of infants born to control mothers under 160.2 cm (63 in.) were 51 cm or more in length; the difference between the two percentages is statistically significant, p< 0.001. Infants with

TABLE 6-4.—DISTRIBUTION OF FULL-TERM INFANTS BORN TO MOTHERS WITH BEHAVIORAL CONDITIONS* ACCORDING TO THEIR OCCIPITOFRONTAL CIRCUMFERENCES AND TO THEIR MOTHERS' HEIGHTS

| MATERNAL HEIGHT | | Total infants No. | OCCIPITOFRONTAL CIRCUMFERENCES (CM) OF FULL-TERM INFANTS | | | | | | Not measured No. |
Cm	In.		≥ 35 No.	%	34.9–33.0 No.	%	< 33 No.	%	
>170.4	(≥67)	187	73	39.0	100	53.5	14	7.5	0
165.3–170.3	(65–66.9)	180	75	41.7	90	50.0	13	7.2	2
160.2–165.2	(63–64.9)	185	64	34.6	101	54.6	19	10.3	1
155.1–160.1	(61–62.9)	178	45	25.3	108	60.7	24	13.5	1
<155.1	(<61)	106	17	16.0	75	70.7	14	13.2	0
Total		836	274	32.8	474	56.7	84	10.0	4

*Behavioral conditions same as in Table 6-2. Mothers with behavioral conditions had none of the other growth-retarding factors in their pregnancies listed in Table 3-1.

crown-heel lengths below 51 cm were more frequently born to mothers under 160.2 cm (63 in.) in height than to taller women.

A more marked effect of maternal height on crown-heel length was observed among mothers with behavioral conditions in their pregnancies (Table 6–2); they had more short infants than did control mothers. In the group of 836 mothers with behavioral conditions, 46.5% of all infants had crown-heel lengths of 51 cm or more, compared to an incidence of 69.5% among all infants born to the 868 control mothers shown in Table 6-1; the difference between the two percentages is statistically significant, p < 0.001. Sixteen per cent of the 836 infants born to women with behavioral conditions had crown-heel lengths under 49 cm, compared to an incidence of 6.2% among the 868 infants born to control mothers shown in Table 6–1; the difference between the two percentages is statistically significant, p< 0.001.

The effect of maternal heights on head circumferences followed the same general patterns as noted in the case of crown-heel lengths (Tables 6–3 and 6–4). In Table 6–3, 48.4% of infants born to control mothers had head circumferences $\geq$ 35 cm, compared to 32.8% of infants born to mothers with behavioral conditions (Table 6–4). In Table 6–3, 5.4% of infants born to control mothers had head circumferences < 33 cm, compared to an incidence of 10% of infants born to mothers with behavioral conditions (Table 6–4). There was a general tendency for short infants to have smaller head circumferences than did long infants, but there were exceptions, particularly among infants born to mothers with behavioral conditions. Most short infants had head circumferences that were appropriate for their gestational ages. A few short infants had head circumferences that were disproportionately large for their crown-heel lengths.

TABLE 6-5.–INCIDENCE OF PREMATURE BIRTHS
(< 37 WEEKS) ACCORDING TO MATERNAL HEIGHT
AND BEHAVIORAL CONDITIONS OF PREGNANCY

MATERNAL HEIGHT		NO BEHAVIORAL CONDITIONS			BEHAVIORAL CONDITIONS[*]		
		Total infants	Premature infants		Total infants	Premature infants	
Cm	In.	No.	No.	%	No.	No.	%
≥170.4	(≥67)	200	4	2.0	200	13	6.5
165.3–170.3	(65–66.9)	200	5	2.5	200	20	10.0
160.2–165.2	(63–64.9)	200	5	2.5	200	15	7.5
155.1–160.1	(61–62.9)	189	2	1.1	191	13	6.8
<155.1	(<61)	99	4	4.0	118	12	10.2
Total		888	20	2.3	909	73	8.0

[*]Behavioral conditions same as in Table 6-2.

TABLE 6-6.—INCIDENCE OF FULL-TERM INFANTS WITH
LOW PONDERAL INDICES (LPI*) ACCORDING TO
MATERNAL HEIGHT AND BEHAVIORAL CONDITIONS
OF PREGNANCY

MATERNAL HEIGHT		NO BEHAVIORAL CONDITIONS			BEHAVIORAL† CONDITIONS		
			Infants			Infants	
		Total	LPI		Total	LPI	
Cm	In.	No.	No.	%	No.	No.	%
≥170.4	(≥67)	196	12	6.1	187	17	9.1
165.3–170.3	(65–66.9)	195	10	5.1	180	13	7.2
160.2–165.2	(63–64.9)	195	10	5.1	185	12	6.5
155.1–160.1	(61–62.9)	187	6	3.2	178	10	5.6
<155.1	(<61)	95	6	6.3	106	8	7.5
Total		868	44	5.1	836	60	7.2

*LPI, below fifth percentile (2.26) for gestational age, based on Rohrer's formula. See Table 4-5.
†Behavioral conditions same as in Table 6-2.

Maternal height had no statistically significant effect on the incidence of premature births among either control mothers or mothers with behavioral conditions (Table 6–5). The incidences of premature births were not significantly different between tall and short mothers. The incidence of premature births was greater among women with behavioral conditions of all different heights than among control mothers of comparable heights.

Full-term infants with low ponderal indices (LPI) were born to control mothers of different heights with frequencies that were not significantly different (Table 6–6). The same lack of significance in incidences of LPI infants was observed among infants born to mothers who had behavioral conditions in their pregnancies and were of different heights.

There was a positive association between maternal height and the incidence of full-term short-for-dates infants among both control mothers and mothers with behavioral conditions in their pregnancies (Table 6–7). The incidences of SHFD infants in Table 6–7 are based on the total number of full-term births. It should be realized that the diagnosis of a SHFD infant depends on knowing the infant's gestational age; 12–15% of white mothers did not know or were uncertain of their pregnancy dates. The differences in incidences of SHFD infants in Table 6–7 could

TABLE 6-7.—INCIDENCE OF FULL-TERM
SHORT-FOR-DATES (SHFD) INFANTS ACCORDING
TO MATERNAL HEIGHT AND PRESENCE OF BEHAVIORAL
CONDITIONS IN MOTHERS

MATERNAL HEIGHT		NO BEHAVIORAL CONDITIONS			BEHAVIORAL° CONDITIONS		
		Total infants	SHFD† infants		Total infants	SHFD† infants	
Cm	In.	No.	No.	%	No.	No.	%
≥170.4	(≥67)	196	3	1.5	187	14	7.5
165.3–170.3	(65–66.9)	195	9	4.6	180	19	10.6
160.2–165.2	(63–64.9)	195	8	4.1	185	32	17.3
155.1–160.1	(61–62.9)	187	23	12.3	178	38	21.3
<155.1	(<61)	95	8	8.4	106	33	31.5
Total		868	51	5.9	836	136	16.3

°Behavioral conditions same as in Table 6-2.
†SHFD, short-for-dates (crown-heel lengths ≤ fifth percentile in Tables 4-2 and 4-3).

not be accounted for by differences in the number of mothers who were uncertain of their pregnancy dates. There were significantly more SHFD infants born to mothers with behavioral conditions than to control mothers. In both the control group of mothers and in the group of mothers with behavioral conditions, the incidence of SHFD infants increased significantly among the shorter mothers. The incidence of SHFD infants was 1.5% among tall control mothers (≥170.4 cm, 67 in.) and 8.4% among short control mothers (<155.1 cm, 61 in.). The difference is significant by the Z test, $p < 0.01$. The trend was similar among mothers with behavioral conditions; the incidence of SHFD infants was 7.5% among tall mothers (≥ 170.4 cm) and 31.5% among short mothers (<155.1 cm). The difference is significant, $p < 0.01$.

The effect of maternal height on the incidence of full-term infants with small occipitofrontal circumferences is shown by data in Table 6–8. Among control mothers, differences in maternal heights did not appear to have a significant association with the incidences of infants with small OF circumferences, but in the group of mothers with behavioral conditions, a significant difference did appear. The incidence of infants with small OF circumferences was 3.7% among tall mothers (≥170.4 cm, 67 in.) and

TABLE 6-8.—INCIDENCE OF FULL-TERM INFANTS WITH
SMALL OCCIPITOFRONTAL (OF) CIRCUMFERENCES
ACCORDING TO MATERNAL HEIGHT AND PRESENCE OF
BEHAVIORAL CONDITIONS IN MOTHERS

MATERNAL HEIGHT		NO BEHAVIORAL CONDITIONS			BEHAVIORAL° CONDITIONS		
		Total infants	Infants with small OF†		Total infants	Infants with small OF†	
Cm	In.	No.	No.	%	No.	No.	%
≥170.4	(≥67)	196	5	2.6	187	7	3.7
165.3–170.3	(65–66.9)	195	8	4.1	180	13	7.2
160.2–165.2	(63–64.9)	195	12	6.2	185	15	8.1
155.1–160.1	(61–62.9)	187	9	4.8	178	17	9.6
<155.1	(<61)	95	6	6.3	106	19	17.9
Total		868	40	4.6	836	71	8.5

°Behavioral conditions same as in Table 6-2.
†Small OF circumferences (≤ fifth percentile, Tables 4-7 and 4-8).

was 17.9% among short mothers (<155.1 cm, 61 in.). The difference is significant, p <0.01.

Low birth weight infants.—Premature infants and full-term SHFD infants were born with greater frequencies to mothers with behavioral conditions than to control mothers, as shown in Tables 6–5 and 6–7, respectively. In Table 6–9, the percentages of low birth weight premature infants, 79.5%, and of SHFD infants, 11.8%, were significantly higher in the group of mothers with behavioral conditions than the respective percentages of 55% and 2% in the group of control mothers. The differences are significant, p < 0.05 in each instance. Almost 80% of the premature infants born to mothers with behavioral conditions had LBW, compared to 55% of premature infants born to control mothers. Likewise, full-term infants with LPIs or who were SHFD were more likely to have LBW if their mothers had behavioral conditions. The heights of mothers had no significant effect on the incidences of LBW infants in either the control groups or groups of mothers who had behavioral conditions.

The association between maternal height and fetal size, as measured by crown-heel length and occipitofrontal circumference, needs to be taken into account in evaluating fetal growth,

TABLE 6-9.—INCIDENCES OF LOW BIRTH WEIGHT (LBW) INFANTS (< 2500 GM) AMONG CONTROL MOTHERS COMPARED TO MOTHERS WITH BEHAVIORAL CONDITIONS

	INFANTS								
	Premature			Full-term					
				LPI†			SHFD‡		
MOTHERS	Total No.	LBW No.	LBW %	Total No.	LBW No.	LBW %	Total No.	LBW No.	LBW %
No behavioral conditions (controls)	20	11	55.0	44	1	2.3	51	1	2.0
Behavioral conditions*	73	58	79.5	60	5	8.3	136	16	11.8

*Behavioral conditions same as in Table 6-2.
†LPI, low ponderal index (< fifth percentile, Table 4-5).
‡SHFD, short-for-dates (≤ fifth percentile, Tables 4-7 and 4-3).

especially in infants born to mothers with behavioral conditions. The same need arises if birth weight is used to evaluate fetal size instead of external body dimensions. In comparing fetal growth between groups of infants, an estimate of the number of short mothers in each group can be made and proper allowance made for any significant skewness in the number of short women.

Otherwise, different standards of fetal growth will be needed for infants of mothers of different heights. The latter could be difficult to obtain, unless the population of short mothers with no other known growth-retarding factors in their pregnancies is large.

REFERENCES

1. Ounsted, M., and Ounsted, C.: *On Fetal Growth Rate: Its Variations and Their Consequences.* Clinics in Developmental Medicine No. 46. Spastics International Medical Publications (London: William Heinemann Medical Books Ltd.; Philadelphia: J. B. Lippincott Company, 1973).

2. The Collaborative Perinatal Study of the National Institutes of Neurological Disease and Stroke: The Women and Their Pregnancies. Department of Health, Education, and Welfare Publication No. (NIH) 73-379, Washington, D. C., U. S. Department of Health, Education, and Welfare, 1972.

7 / Prepregnancy Maternal Habitus (Weight for Height)

THE EFFECT of prepregnancy maternal weight on fetal growth has been studied in two different ways. Some investigators have used maternal weight by itself and others have preferred a weight-for-height standard. Pregnancy outcome for the fetus depends on which of these two methods is used. To say that a woman who weighs less than 54.5 kg (120 lb) is underweight does not appropriately characterize all women who weigh less than 54.5 kg. According to Sargent's table for young women, an individual who is 150 cm tall (59 in.) and weighs 54 kg (119 lb) is overweight for her height.[1] A weight-for-height standard comes nearer to describing an individual's body build and nutritional state; consequently, we have used a weight-for-height standard.[1] In determining the weight for height of each gravida, we relied on her statement as to what her prepregnancy weight was. Some women did not know their prepregnancy weights and they were either excluded altogether from the study or admitted with an appropriate note to the exception. Women who had no prenatal care were particularly unlikely to know their prepregnancy or pregnancy weights.

Previous investigators observed a positive relationship between the prepregnancy weights of mothers and their infants' birth weights.[2-8] Data in Table 4–14 of this study reveal a similar relationship; mothers who were above average in their weight-height ratio at conception had heavier babies than did mothers who were below average. This positive relationship between birth weight and the prepregnancy habitus of the mother did not appear to depend on an increase in crown-heel lengths of infants, judging by the data in Table 4–4. However, as seen in Table 4–9, occipitofrontal circumferences tended to be larger in overweight mothers than in underweight mothers; this relationship is important in interpreting the data in Table 7–4, showing a tenfold increase in births of infants with small head circumferences among underweight mothers as compared to obese mothers.

Data in this chapter are limited to infants of control mothers of different prepregnancy habitus. The control mothers had none of the other growth-retarding factors in their pregnancies listed in Table 3–1, so far as could be judged from a review of their medical and obstetric records and from a personal interview with each mother obtained by the senior author before the mothers and babies were discharged from The University of Kansas Medical Center.

The prepregnancy habitus of control mothers had no significant effect on the incidence of premature births (Table 7–1). Few premature infants were born to control mothers in any of the maternal weight-height groups. The over-all incidence of premature births was 2.4%.

According to the definitions used in this study, one would expect that about 5% of full-term infants born to control mothers would have low ponderal indices (LPI), about 5% would be short-for-dates (SHFD) and about 5% would have small oc-

TABLE 7-1.—INCIDENCE OF PREMATURE INFANTS
(< 37 COMPLETED WEEKS OF GESTATION)
ACCORDING TO MATERNAL PREPREGNANCY
HABITUS OF CONTROL MOTHERS

MATERNAL WEIGHT FOR HEIGHT°	NO FETAL GROWTH-RETARDING FACTORS (CONTROLS)		
	Total infants	Premature infants Total	
	No.	No.	%
Obese, > 30% above normal°	121	3	2.5
Overweight, 7.5–30% above normal	353	10	2.8
Average weight for height†	650	18	2.8
Slender, 7.5–15% below normal	240	3	1.3
Underweight, ≥ 15% below normal	70	1	1.4
Total	1434	35	2.4

°Based on Sargent's table for young women.[1]
†From 7.5% above to 7.5% below normal.

TABLE 7-2.—INCIDENCE OF BIRTHS OF
FULL-TERM INFANTS WITH LOW PONDERAL
INDICES (LPI)* ACCORDING TO MATERNAL
PREPREGNANCY HABITUS OF CONTROL
MOTHERS

MATERNAL WEIGHT FOR HEIGHT†	NO FETAL GROWTH-RETARDING FACTORS (CONTROLS)		
	Total infants	LPI full-term infants Total	
	No.	No.	%
Obese, > 30% above normal†	118	3	2.5
Overweight, 7.5–30% above normal	343	17	4.9
Average weight for height‡	632	28	4.3
Slender, 7.5–15% below normal	237	14	5.9
Underweight, ≥ 15% below normal	69	4	5.8
Total	1399	66	4.7

*LPI, < fifth percentile, Table 4-5.
†Based on Sargent's table for young women.[1]
‡From 7.5% above to 7.5% below normal.

cipitofrontal circumferences. In Table 7–2, the over-all incidence of infants with low ponderal indices was 4.7% among full-term infants born to 1399 control mothers. The prepregnancy habitus of the mothers did not appear to affect the incidence of LPI full-term infants significantly. The incidence of LPI infants among 118 obese women was 2.5%, but the number of LPI infants was too few to attach statistical significance to this observation.

The incidence of full-term SHFD infants among control mothers in Table 7–3 followed a pattern similar to that in Table 7–2. The over-all incidence was 6.1% among 1399 full-term infants and was not significantly above the expected incidence of 5% based on definition. As in Table 7–2, obese women had fewer SHFD infants than did women in the lower weight-height groups. As with the LPI full-term infants, the number of SHFD full-term infants born to obese mothers was too few for statistical analysis.

The effect of prepregnancy habitus of control mothers on occipitofrontal circumferences of their infants was marked (Table

TABLE 7-3.—INCIDENCE OF BIRTHS OF FULL-TERM
SHORT-FOR-DATES (SHFD*) INFANTS ACCORDING
TO MATERNAL PREPREGNANCY HABITUS OF
CONTROL MOTHERS

| MATERNAL WEIGHT FOR HEIGHT† | NO FETAL GROWTH-RETARDING FACTORS (CONTROLS) | | |
| | Total infants | SHFD full-term infants Total | |
	No.	No.	%
Obese, > 30% above normal†	118	5	4.4
Overweight, 7.5–30% above normal	343	25	7.3
Average weight for height‡	632	30	4.8
Slender, 7.5–15% below normal	237	19	8.0
Underweight, ≥ 15% below normal	69	6	8.7
Total	1399	85	6.1

*SHFD, ≤ fifth percentile, Tables 4-2 and 4-3.
†Based on Sargent's table for young women.[1]
‡From 7.5% above to 7.5% below normal.

TABLE 7-4.—INCIDENCE OF BIRTHS OF
FULL-TERM INFANTS WITH SMALL
OCCIPITOFRONTAL (OF)* CIRCUMFERENCES
ACCORDING TO MATERNAL PREPREGNANCY
HABITUS OF CONTROL MOTHERS

| MATERNAL WEIGHT FOR HEIGHT† | NO FETAL GROWTH-RETARDING FACTORS (CONTROLS) | | |
| | Total infants | Small OF full-term infants Total | |
	No.	No.	%
Obese, > 30% above normal†	118	1	0.8
Overweight, 7.5–30% above normal	343	8	2.3
Average weight for height‡	632	27	4.3
Slender, 7.5–15% below normal	237	23	9.7
Underweight, ≥ 15% below normal	69	6	8.7
Total	1399	65	4.6

*OF circumferences, ≤ fifth percentile, Tables 4-7 and 4-8.
†Based on Sargent's table for young women.[1]
‡From 7.5% above to 7.5% below normal.

7 – 4). The over-all incidence of infants with small OF circumferences was 4.6% and was well within the expected range of 5% for infants of control mothers. However, there was a tenfold difference between obese and underweight mothers. The incidence of infants with small OF circumferences was low (0.8%) among obese mothers and rose significantly to an incidence of 9.7% among infants of slender mothers and to 8.7% among infants of underweight mothers. The differences between the low and the two high incidences are significant by the Z test, $p < 0.01$ in each instance. This strong relationship between prepregnancy habitus of the mothers and the incidence of full-term infants with small head circumferences was also observed among mothers who had behavioral conditions in their pregnancy, as shown in Table 8 – 3 in the next chapter.

The association of an increased incidence of infants with small OF circumferences among slender and underweight mothers is a new observation and one not previously reported in the literature, so far as we know. It has implication for sonographers who are judging fetal maturity and size by measuring biparietal diameters with ultrasound techniques. It may have additional implications for postnatal growth and development. Further study of the relationship between maternal prepregnancy habitus and head size of infants is warranted.

Low birth weight infants. – There was no evidence that differences in maternal prepregnancy habitus of control mothers were associated with significant differences in the incidences of LBW infants, in either premature or full-term infants.

REFERENCES
1. Sargent, D. W.: Weight-height relationship of young men and women, Am. J. Clin. Nutr. 13:318, 1963.
2. Tompkins, W. T., Wiehl, D. G., and Mitchell, R. McN.: The underweight patient as an increased obstetric hazard, Am. J. Obstet. Gynecol. 69:114, 1955.
3. Eastman, N. J., and Jackson, E.: Weight relationships in pregnancy, Obstet. Gynecol. Surv. 21:1003, 1968.
4. Niswander, K. R., Singer, J., Westphal, M., and Weiss, W.: Weight gain during pregnancy and pregnancy weight, Obstet. Gynecol. 33: 482, 1969.
5. Love, E. J., and Kinch, R. A. H.: Factors influencing the birth weight in normal pregnancy, Am. J. Obstet. Gynecol. 91:342, 1965.
6. Weiss, W., and Jackson, E. C.: Maternal factors affecting birth weight, Proc. Pan-Am. Health Org., October, 1969.

7. Niswander, K., and Jackson, E. C.: Physical characteristics of the gravida and their association with birth weight and perinatal death, Am. J. Obstet. Gynecol. 119:306, 1974.

8. The Collaborative Perinatal Study of the National Institutes of Neurological Disease and Stroke: The Women and Their Pregnancies. Department of Health, Education, and Welfare Publication No. (NIH) 73-379, Washington, D. C., U. S. Department of Health, Education, and Welfare, 1972.

8 / Low Weight Gains in Pregnancy

THERE IS GENERAL AGREEMENT that a strong positive relationship exists between the amount of maternal weight gained in pregnancy and birth weight of offspring.[1-5] Particular interest in this chapter centers on the effects of low weight gains (LWG). Next to cigarette smoking, LWG has been the most frequently observed behavioral condition, occurring in 15–20% of women delivered at The University of Kansas Medical Center.

Two basic questions arise in connection with maternal weight gains. How should weight gain be determined and what constitutes a LWG? We have relied on weight gained in the last two trimesters, because that was when gravidas gained the most weight and when their weights obtained at prenatal visits were likely to have been recorded. Weight gains for the total duration of pregnancy depended on women knowing their prepregnancy weights; many of them could not provide reliable recollections of their weights, especially women in the lower socioeconomic groups. Errors by mothers in estimating their prepregnancy weights possibly account for the paradoxical observation in the study of 25,000 pregnancies at Johns Hopkins Hospital by Eastman and Jackson, in which the mean birth weight of infants born to white mothers with negative weight gains was greater than the mean birth weights of infants born to mothers who gained 0–10 pounds or 11–20 pounds in their pregnancies.[1]

We have arbitrarily defined a LWG as a mean weight gain of 227 gm (½ lb) or less per week in the last two trimesters. Women are said to gain on the average 1 kg (2 lb) in the first trimester and 5 kg (11 lb) in each of the last two trimesters for a total of about 11 kg or about 24 lb.[6] The combined weight of the products of conception, including fetus, placenta, amniotic fluid and increase in weight of the uterus, breasts and extra blood volume, is said to be about 8 kg in an average term pregnancy.[6] The upper limit of the low weight gain used in the present study, 227 gm per week during the last two trimesters, comes to a total of about 6 kg. Adding 1 kg gained in the first trimester would bring the total to 7 kg, which is less than the total average weight of the products of conception at term (40 weeks). In practice, our definition of a LWG has been satisfactory in making statistical evaluations on large numbers of women and their offspring. Data to be presented in this chapter clearly indicate, however, that the effects of LWG on infants born at The University of Kansas Medical Center depended to a considerable extent on the mothers' prepregnancy weights. Pregnancy outcome for fetuses of underweight women was poorer than for women whose prepregnancy weights were average or above average for their heights.

About 20% of white mothers delivered at this Medical Center during the present study had less than 10 weeks of prenatal care prior to delivery. In such mothers, weight gains in pregnancy were not calculated on weights recorded at prenatal visits but on total weight gained in the last two trimesters. The latter weight gain was calculated by subtracting 3 lb from the total weight gained in pregnancy to allow for weight gained in the first trimester and then dividing the remainder by the duration of pregnancy in weeks in the last two trimesters.

In general, about 70% of white women with LWG in the present study were multipara and tended to have average or better than average weights for their heights at conception, an observation that is in keeping with reports by previous investigators. LWG were also about 3 times more frequent among women in the lowest than among those in the highest socioeconomic group. Women in the lowest socioeconomic group were more likely to be *overweight* at conception than women in the highest socioeconomic group.

White women in this study who had LWG in their pregnancies had more premature infants and more births of undergrown full-term infants than did control mothers who were judged to have none of the growth-retarding factors in their pregnancies listed in Table 3–1. Premature births increased significantly from a low of 2.4% among control mothers to 10.4% among mothers with LWG (Table 8–1). There were increased births of premature infants among mothers with LWG who also smoked ciga-

TABLE 8-1.—INCIDENCES OF PREMATURE INFANTS
(< 37 COMPLETED WEEKS OF GESTATION) AMONG
MOTHERS WITH LOW WEIGHT GAINS (LWG)
IN PREGNANCY COMPARED TO CONTROL MOTHERS

MOTHERS WITH LWG° IN PREGNANCY		PREMATURE INFANTS	
	No.	No.	%
Mothers with			
LWG only	118	7	5.9
LWG and cigarette smoking	129	13	10.0
LWG, smoking and other behaviors†	31	6	19.3
LWG and other behaviors†	20	5	25.0
Total mothers with LWG	298	31	10.4
Control mothers‡	1434	35	2.4

°LWG, ≤227 gm per week in last two trimesters.
†Other behaviors included delivery before seventeenth or after thirty-fifth birthdays, use of addicting drugs or chronic alcoholism, being underweight at conception and no prenatal care. See group III, Table 3-1.
‡Control mothers had none of the growth-retarding factors in Table 3-1.

rettes during pregnancy or had other behavioral conditions in their pregnancies. Premature births were 5.9% among women whose only behavioral condition was a LWG and increased to 10% among women with LWG who also smoked cigarettes and to 19.3% among women with LWG who smoked cigarettes and had other behavioral conditions. The combination of a LWG with cigarette smoking occurred in more than 40% of mothers with LWG and was observed more frequently than a LWG by itself.

The incidence of full-term infants with low ponderal indices (LPI) and the incidence of full-term short-for-dates (SHFD) were greater among women with LWG than among control mothers (Table 8–2). The incidence of full-term infants with LPI among mothers with LWG was 11.6% and among control mothers the incidence was 4.5%. The difference is significant by the Z test, $p < 0.01$. SHFD infants increased from 6.1% among control mothers to 16.8% among mothers with LWG. The difference is significant, $p < 0.01$. The incidence of SHFD infants was higher among mothers who had LWG and other behavioral conditions than it was among mothers who just had a LWG without other known

TABLE 8-2.—INCIDENCES OF UNDERGROWN FULL-TERM INFANTS BORN TO MOTHERS WITH LOW WEIGHT GAINS (LWG) IN PREGNANCY COMPARED TO CONTROL MOTHERS

MOTHERS WITH LWG§ IN PREGNANCY	No.	UNDERGROWN FULL-TERM INFANTS					
		LPI*		SHFD†		Small OF‡	
		No.	%	No.	%	No.	%
Mothers with							
LWG only	111	14	12.6	12	10.8	6	5.5
LWG and cigarette smoking	116	13	11.2	25	20.8	11	9.5
LWG, smoking and other behaviors‖	25	3	12.0	3	12.0	2	8.0
LWG and other behaviors‖	15	1	6.7	5	33.0	1	6.7
Total mothers with LWG	267	31	11.6	45	16.8	20	7.5
Control mothers	1399	65	4.5	85	6.1	65	4.5

*LPI, low ponderal index (< fifth percentile, Table 4-5).
†SHFD, short-for-dates (≤ fifth percentile, Tables 4-2 and 4-3).
‡Small OF, occipitofrontal circumferences (≤ fifth percentile, Tables 4-7 and 4-8).
§LWG, ≤ 227 gm per week, last two trimesters.
‖Other behaviors, see Table 8-1.

TABLE 8-3.– PREGNANCY OUTCOME AMONG MOTHERS WITH LOW WEIGHT GAINS (LWG) IN PREGNANCY ACCORDING TO THEIR PREPREGNANCY HABITUS

MATERNAL* WEIGHT-HEIGHT RATIO, PREPREGNANCY	TOTAL INFANTS No.	PREMATURE INFANTS (< 37 WKS) No.	%	FULL-TERM INFANTS							
				Total No.	LPI‡ No.	%	SHFD§ No.	%	OF‖ circs. No.	%
≥ 7.5% above normal*	172	12	7.0	160	15	9.4	19	11.9	7	4.4
Average†	82	6	7.3	76	11	14.5	14	18.4	9	11.8
≥ 7.5% below normal	44	13	29.5	31	5	16.1	12	38.7	4	12.9

*Based on Sargent's table for young women.[7]
†From 7.5% above to 7.5% below normal in Sargent's table.[7]
‡LPI, low ponderal index (< fifth percentile, Table 4-5).
§SHFD, short-for-dates (≤ fifth percentile, Tables 4-2 and 4-3).
‖OF circs., occipitofrontal circumferences (≤ fifth percentile, Tables 4-7 and 4-8).

TABLE 8-4.—INCIDENCE OF LOW BIRTH WEIGHT (LBW)
INFANTS (< 2500 GM) AMONG CONTROL MOTHERS
AND MOTHERS WITH LOW WEIGHT GAINS (LWG)

		INFANTS					
		Premature			Full-term		
MOTHERS		(< 37 weeks)					
		Total	LBW		Total	LBW	
	No.	No.	No.	%	No.	No.	%
Control mothers	1434	35	21	60.0	150	7	4.7
Mothers with LWG	298	31	29	93.5	76	10	13.2

growth-retarding factors in their pregnancies. There was a slight
but not significant increase of infants with small occipitofrontal
circumferences born to mothers with LWG.

The combination of LWG with a low prepregnancy habitus
was associated with a particularly poor pregnancy outcome
(Table 8–3). In the latter group of women, the incidence of premature births was 29.5% as compared to 7% among women with
average or above average prepregnancy habitus. The incidence
of full-term SHFD infants among women who were underweight
at conception and had LWG was 38.7% and was 3 times higher
than among mothers who were overweight and had LWG. Overweight women who had LWG had the lowest incidences of full-
term infants with low ponderal indices or with small occipitofrontal circumferences.

The proportion of premature infants and of undergrown full-
term infants who had low birth weights was higher among wom-
en with LWG than among control mothers (Table 8–4). The incidence of LBW premature infants was 60% among premature infants born to control mothers and 93.5% among premature infants born to mothers with LWG; 4.7% of undergrown full-term
infants born to control mothers had low birth weights and 13.2%
of undergrown full-term infants born to mothers with LWG had
low birth weights.

REFERENCES

1. Eastman, N. J., and Jackson, E.: Weight relationships in pregnancy,
   Obstet. Gynecol. Surv. 21:1003, 1968.
2. Singer, J. E., Westphal, M., and Niswander, K.: Relationship of

weight gain in pregnancy to birth weight and infant growth and development in the first year of life, Obstet. Gynecol. 31:417, 1968.

3. Niswander, K. R., Singer, J., Westphal, M., and Weiss, W.: Weight gain during pregnancy and prepregnancy weight, Obstet. Gynecol. 33:482, 1969.

4. Love, E. J., and Kinch, R. A. H.: Factors influencing the birth weight in normal pregnancy, Am. J. Obstet. Gynecol. 91:342, 1965.

5. Weiss, W., and Jackson, E. C.: Maternal factors affecting birth weight, Proc. Pan-Am. Health Org., October, 1969.

6. Pritchard, J. A., and MacDonald, P. C.: *Williams' Obstetrics* (15th ed.; New York: Appleton Century-Crofts, 1976).

7. Sargent, D. W.: Weight-height relationship of young men and women, Am. J. Clin. Nutr. 13:318, 1963.

8. Miller, H. C., and Hassanein, K.: Fetal malnutrition in white newborn infants: Maternal factors, Pediatrics 52:504, 1973.

9. Miller, H. C., and Hassanein, K.: Maternal factors in "fetally malnourished" black newborn infants, Am. J. Obstet. Gynecol. 118:62, 1974.

10. Miller, H. C., and Hassanein, K.: Maternal smoking and fetal growth of full-term infants, Pediatr. Res. 8:960, 1974.

9 / White Teenage Pregnancies

MUCH HAS BEEN WRITTEN about pregnancy outcome among teenagers. Most investigators have reported a high incidence of premature births and an associated increase in neonatal mortality.[1-10] It is not clear from these previous reports how much of the increase in premature births was related to a youthful maternal age and how much to other factors so frequently mentioned in teenage pregnancies, such as lack of prenatal care, poor eating habits, poor nutrition, cigarette smoking and, according to some investigators, an unusually high incidence of medical complications of pregnancy. Differences in pregnancy outcome might also be expected between very young and older teenagers and between primiparas and multiparas. In this chapter, white teenagers delivered consecutively at The University of Kansas Medical Center have been grouped according to their ages, parity and the occurrence of medical complications of pregnancy listed under group II, Table 3–1, and the presence of seven behavioral conditions listed under group III of the same table.

White teenagers as a group compared favorably with white mothers of all ages. For example, the incidence of white mothers of all ages with medical complications of pregnancy, as shown in Table 5–1, was 15%. In the combined group of 770 primiparous and multiparous teenagers in Tables 9–1 and 9–2 it was 15.4%. Forty-five per cent of all white mothers of all ages in Table 5–1 had behavioral conditions in their pregnancies; the incidence of primiparous teenagers who had behavioral conditions (Table 9–1) was 47.3%. Multiparous teenagers in Table 9–2 had a higher incidence of gravidas with behavioral conditions (55%). The incidence of white mothers of all ages who had no known growth-retarding factors in their pregnancies was 39% in Table 5–1 and in teenagers in Tables 9–1 and 9–2 it was about 35%.

Teenagers with medical complications of pregnancy were not observed more frequently in the age range under 17 years than

TABLE 9-1.—DISTRIBUTION OF TEENAGE PRIMIPARAS WITH MEDICAL
COMPLICATIONS OF PREGNANCY AND MATERNAL BEHAVIORAL
CONDITIONS ACCORDING TO THEIR AGES

MATERNAL AGE AT DELIVERY (YEARS)	MOTHERS WITH MEDICAL COMPLICATIONS[*] No.	%	MOTHERS WITH BEHAVIORAL CONDITIONS[†] No.	%	MOTHERS WITH NO KNOWN GROWTH-RETARDING FACTORS[‡] No.	%	TOTAL MOTHERS No.	%
19	28	16.8	73	43.7	66	39.5	167	100.0
18	16	10.7	77	51.3	57	38.0	150	100.0
17	26	18.8	64	46.4	48	34.8	138	100.0
16	25	22.3	56	50.0	31	27.7	112	100.0
15	5	11.1	20	44.5	20	44.5	45	100.0
≤14	5	38.5	6	46.1	2	15.4	13	100.0
Total	105	16.8	296	47.3	224	35.9	625	100.0

[*]Medical complications listed in group II, Table 3-1.
[†]Behavioral conditions listed in group III, Table 3-1.
[‡]None of the factors listed in Table 3-1.

in older teenagers, either among primiparas in Table 9-1, or among multiparas in Table 9-2, except in the small group of 13 primiparous teenagers under 15 years of age. In this small group, there were 5 teenagers who had medical complications, 4 of whom had preeclampsia. Behavioral conditions in teenage preg-

TABLE 9-2.—DISTRIBUTION OF TEENAGE MULTIPARAS WITH MEDICAL
COMPLICATIONS OF PREGNANCY AND MATERNAL BEHAVIORAL
CONDITIONS ACCORDING TO THEIR AGES

MATERNAL AGE AT DELIVERY (YEARS)	MOTHERS WITH MEDICAL COMPLICATIONS°		MOTHERS WITH BEHAVIORAL CONDITIONS†		MOTHERS WITH NO KNOWN GROWTH-RETARDING FACTORS‡		TOTAL MOTHERS	
	No.	%	No.	%	No.	%	No.	%
19	8	10.0	43	53.7	29	36.3	80	100.0
18	4	10.8	20	54.1	13	35.1	37	100.0
17	0	0.0	11	73.4	4	26.6	15	100.0
16	2	15.4	6	46.1	5	38.5	13	100.0
Total	14	9.6	80	55.2	51	35.2	145	100.0

°Medical complications listed in group II, Table 3-1.
†Behavioral conditions listed in group III, Table 3-1.
‡None of the factors listed in Table 3-1.

nancies were not seen more frequently in those under 17 years of age at delivery than in those 17 years or over. Except in the group of primiparas under 15 years of age, the incidences of mothers with no known growth-retarding factors in their pregnancies were not significantly different among teenagers whose

TABLE 9–3.—PREGNANCY OUTCOME AMONG WHITE PRIMIPAROUS CONTROL MOTHERS ACCORDING TO MATERNAL AGE

MATERNAL AGE AT DELIVERY (YEARS)	TOTAL INFANTS No.	PREMATURE INFANTS (< 37 WEEKS)		FULL-TERM INFANTS							
		No.	%	Total No.	LPI° No.	%	SHFD† No.	%	Small OF‡ circ. No.	%
19–17	171	7	4.1	164	7	4.3	7	4.3	5	3.2
≤ 16	53	4	7.5	49	2	4.2	8	16.3	2	4.2
Total teenagers	224	11	4.9	213	9	4.2	15	7.0	7	3.3
34–20	384	9	2.3	375	21	5.6	29	7.7	18	4.8

°LPI, low ponderal index (< fifth percentile, Table 4-5).
†SHFD, short-for-dates (≤ fifth percentile, Tables 4-2 and 4-3).
‡Small OF, occipitofrontal circumferences (≤ fifth percentile, Tables 4-7 and 4-8).

ages ranged from 15 to 19 years. In that small group of teenagers under 15 years of age there were only 2 mothers who had no known growth-retarding factors.

Pregnancy outcome among 224 primiparous teenagers who had no known growth-retarding factors in their pregnancies is shown in Table 9–3 and compared to pregnancy outcome among 384 control primiparas from 20 to 34 years of age. More premature infants were born to 224 teenagers (4.9%) than to the 384 mothers who were 20 or more years of age (2.3%) but the difference was not statistically significant. The 53 teenagers under 17 years of age had a higher incidence of premature infants (7.5%) than 171 teenagers from 17 to 19 years of age (5.1%) but again the difference was not statistically significant. There was a statistically significant difference between the percentage (16.3%) of short-for-dates full-term infants born to primiparous teenagers under 17 years of age and the percentage (4.3%) born to older teenagers. The difference is statistically significant by the chi-square test, $p < 0.01$. Full-term infants with low ponderal indices and small occipitofrontal circumferences were not significantly increased among teenagers from 13 to 19 years of age.

Pregnancy outcome among multiparous teenagers who had no known growth-retarding factors in their pregnancies was limited to 51 mothers who fit the criteria. The group was small. No obvious deviations in premature births or births of undergrown full-term infants were observed.

Pregnancy outcome among primiparas in the teenage group who had behavioral conditions in their pregnancies is shown in Table 9–4. Premature births and births of undergrown full-term infants were not significantly higher among primiparas under 17 years of age than among primiparas from 17 to 19 years of age. Furthermore, the incidences of premature births and of undergrown full-term infants were not significantly higher among primiparous teenagers than among primiparas who ranged in age from 20 to 34 years.

Low birth weight infants. — Most LBW white infants born at The University of Kansas Medical Center had mothers with behavioral conditions and no other known growth-retarding factors in their pregnancies. Teenagers were no exception. There were 54 LBW infants born to teenagers from 13 to 19 years of age and 29 of them were born to teenagers whose mothers had

TABLE 9–4.—PREGNANCY OUTCOME AMONG WHITE PRIMIPARAS WITH BEHAVIORAL CONDITIONS* ACCORDING TO MATERNAL AGE

MATERNAL AGE AT DELIVERY (YEARS)	TOTAL INFANTS No.	PREMATURE INFANTS (< 37 WEEKS)		FULL-TERM INFANTS							
		No.	%	Total No.	LPI† No.	%	SHFD‡ No.	%	Small OF§ circ. No.	%
19–17	214	21	9.8	193	14	7.3	39	21.0	11	5.7
≤ 16	82	7	8.5	75	3	4.0	8	10.7	4	5.3
Total teenagers	296	28	9.5	268	17	6.3	47	17.5	15	5.6
34–20	248	21	8.4	227	18	7.9	32	14.8	17	7.5

*Behavioral conditions, see Table 3-1.
†LPI, low ponderal index (< fifth percentile, Table 4-5).
‡SHFD, short-for-dates (≤ fifth percentile, Tables 4-2 and 4-3).
§Small OF, occipitofrontal circumferences (≤ fifth percentile, Tables 4-7 and 4-8).

TABLE 9-5.—INCIDENCE OF LOW BIRTH WEIGHT (LBW) INFANTS (< 2500 GM) ACCORDING TO MATERNAL AGES OF PRIMIPARAS AND TO PRESENCE OF[1] MEDICAL COMPLICATIONS AND BEHAVIORAL CONDITIONS

MATERNAL AGE AT DELIVERY (YEARS)	NO FETAL GROWTH-RETARDING FACTORS[°]			BEHAVIORAL CONDITIONS[†]			MEDICAL COMPLICATIONS OF PREGNANCY[‡]		
	Mothers No.	LBW infants No.	%	Mothers No.	LBW infants No.	%	Mothers No.	LBW infants No.	%
19–17	171	4	2.3	214	21	9.8	70	9	12.8
16–15	51	3	5.9	76	6	7.8	30	8	26.4
≤14	2	1	50.0	6	2	33.3	5	0	0.0
Total teenagers	224	8	3.6	296	29	9.8	105	17	16.2
34–20	384	8	2.3	248	26	10.5	-	-	-

° None of the growth-retarding factors in Table 3-1.
† Behavioral conditions, group III, Table 3-1.
‡ Medical complications, group II, Table 3-1.

behavioral conditions (Table 9–5). The incidence of LBW infants born to teenagers with behavioral conditions was 9.8% and not significantly higher than the incidence of 10.5% among white primiparas 20–34 years of age. The incidence of LBW infants born to teenagers with no known growth-retarding factors in their pregnancies was 3.6% and was not significantly higher than the incidence of LBW infants (2.3%) born to control primiparas 20–34 years of age. The small group of teenagers under 15 years of age did have higher incidences of LBW infants than older teenagers, but the number of those under 15 years of age was too small to test statistical significance.

REFERENCES

1. Battaglia, F. C., Frazier, T. M., and Hellegers, A. E.: Obstetric and pediatric complications of juvenile pregnancy, Pediatrics 32:902, 1963.
2. Claman, A. D., and Bell, H. M.: Pregnancy in the very young teenager, Am. J. Obstet. Gynecol. 90:350, 1964.
3. Dickens, H. O., et al.: One hundred pregnant adolescents. Treatment approaches in a university hospital, Am. J. Public Health 63: 794, 1973.
4. Klein, L.: Early teenage pregnancy, contraception and repeat pregnancy, Am. J. Obstet. Gynecol. 120:249, 1974.
5. Duenhoelter, J. H., Jimenez, J. M., and Baumann, G.: Pregnancy performance of patients under fifteen years of age, Obstet. Gynecol. 46:49, 1975.
6. Houde, C. T., and Conway, C. E.: Teen-age mothers: A clinical profile, Contemp. Ob/Gyn. 7:71, 1976.
7. Dwyer, J. F.: Teenage pregnancy, Am. J. Obstet. Gynecol. 118:373, 1974.
8. Jekel, J. F., et al.: A comparison of the health of index and subsequent babies born to school age mothers, Am. J. Public Health 65: 370, 1975.
9. McAnarney, E. R., and Friedman, S. B.: Experience with an adolescent health care program, Public Health Rep. 90:412, 1975.
10. McAnarney, E. R., et al.: Obstetric, neonatal and psychosocial outcome of pregnant adolescents, Pediatrics 61:199, 1978.

10 / Maternal Age of 35 Years or More

PREGNANCY OUTCOME for older women is said to be unfavorable as compared to pregnancy outcome among younger women.[1] Mean birth weights are reported to diminish and the incidence of low birth weight infants to increase with advancing age. Data provided in this chapter on white mothers delivered at The University of Kansas Medical Center show that pregnancy outcome is good among women who have passed their thirty-fifth birthday, except for an increased risk of congenital malformations, provided that they have had no complications of pregnancy and none of the other growth-retarding factors in their pregnancies listed in Table 3-1.

There were 116 white mothers who were 35-47 years of age delivered consecutively at The University of Kansas Medical Center. Six of the 116 infants had congenital malformations that were identified at birth; 3 infants had Down's syndrome, 1 infant had a cleft lip and palate and 2 infants had minor defects — a first-degree hypospadias and a lumbar dimple. There was a high degree of fetal growth retardation among the 6 infants. All 6 were full-term infants; 4 infants were short-for-dates and all 4 had small occipitofrontal circumferences (≤fifth percentile for their gestational ages). A fifth infant had a low ponderal index. Four of the 6 mothers had growth-retarding factors in their pregnancies; 3 mothers had low weight gains in their pregnancies and a fourth mother had chronic hypertension.

Data on 110 infants who had no identifiable congenital malformations at birth are shown in Table 10-1. The numbers of mothers are small, but they show distinct differences in premature births and births of short-for-dates full-term infants. The 35 mothers who had no known growth-retarding factors in their pregnancies had no premature births and no short-for-dates full-

TABLE 10–1.—PREGNANCY OUTCOME AMONG WHITE
MOTHERS 35 YEARS OR OLDER

MATERNAL GROWTH-RETARDING FACTORS	TOTAL INFANTS	PREMATURE INFANTS (< 37 WEEKS)		FULL-TERM INFANTS Total	SHFD†	
	No.	No.	%	No.	No.	%
None present	35	0	0.0	35	0	0.0
Medical complications*	31	6	19.4	25	4	8.0
Behavioral* conditions	44	7	15.9	37	10	27.0
Total	110	13	11.8	97	14	14.4

*See Table 3-1.
†SHFD, short-for-dates (≤ fifth percentile, Tables 4-2 and 4-3).

term infants. Mothers with medical complications of pregnancy had a high incidence of premature births (19.4%). Mothers with behavioral conditions in their pregnancies also had a high incidence of premature births (15.9%) and a high incidence of short-for-dates infants (27%). Full-term infants with low ponderal indices were not significantly increased among mothers 35 or more years of age.

The types of behavioral conditions observed in this older age group of women followed the pattern observed among younger women. Cigarette smoking during pregnancy was the most frequent condition and low weight gain in pregnancy was the next most frequent. A surprisingly large number (7 of 116) had no prenatal care.

Low birth weight infants. — No LBW infants were born to the 35 mothers in Table 10-1 who had no known growth-retarding factors in their pregnancies. There were 10 LBW infants born to the 44 mothers with behavioral problems, an incidence of 22.7%, and 6 LBW infants were born to the 31 mothers with medical complications in their pregnancies, an incidence of 19.3%. Thirteen of the 16 LBW infants were born prematurely.

REFERENCE
1. The Collaborative Perinatal Study of the National Institutes of Neurological Disease and Stroke: The Women and Their Pregnancies. Department of Health, Education, and Welfare Publication No. (NIH) 73-379, Washington, D. C., U. S. Department of Health, Education, and Welfare, 1972.

11 / Maternal Cigarette Smoking

NUMEROUS REPORTS have appeared on the risks confronting fetuses whose mothers smoke cigarettes during pregnancy. The list of potential risks for human fetuses is impressive. It includes increased risk of spontaneous abortion,[1] increased early fetal and neonatal deaths associated with abruptio placentae, placenta previa and premature, prolonged rupture of the membranes,[2] significant reduction in mean birth weight,[3, 4] significant reduction in mean body length at birth,[5-7] increased births of premature (< 37 completed weeks of gestation) infants and of low birth weight (< 2500 gm) infants.[8] The teratogenic aspects of maternal cigarette smoking during pregnancy are controversial. The Surgeon General of the United States concluded that the possible teratogenic effects of maternal smoking had not been adequately evaluated.[9] Other reports by the Surgeon General summarize the published studies on the effects of maternal smoking on the fetus up to 1973.[10] The explanation for the reduction in birth weight among infants born to mothers who smoked during pregnancy also appears clouded. Rush[11] suggested that the reduction in birth weight was in part mediated by depressed caloric intake by mothers and that their lower caloric consumption was reflected in a lower maternal weight gain during pregnancy. There is no doubt that some mothers who smoke cigarettes also have poor weight gains during pregnancy. The combined effect of these two behavioral conditions on the fetus is worse than either one appearing alone. Data presented in Tables 8–2 and 8–3 in this text show that the combination of cigarette smoking and a low weight gain in pregnancy was associated with higher incidences of premature births and of short-for-dates infants than the occurrence of a low weight gain by itself. The important fact to recognize is that maternal cigarette smoking unassociated with any other of the growth-retarding factors that are listed in Table 3–1 can be accompanied by an increase in premature births (Table

TABLE 11–1.—INCIDENCES OF
PREMATURE BIRTHS (< 37
COMPLETED WEEKS OF
PREGNANCY) ACCORDING TO
NUMBER OF CIGARETTES SMOKED
PER DAY DURING PREGNANCY BY
GRAVIDAS

NUMBER OF CIGARETTES REPORTED SMOKED PER DAY	INFANTS		
	Total	Premature	
	No.	No.	%
≤ 21	134	11	8.2
11 – 20	285	17	6.0
6 – 10	146	9	6.1
1 – 5	63	2	3.1
0	1434	35	2.4

11 – 1) and by an increase in births of short-for-dates full-term infants (Table 11 – 2). The reduction in birth weight associated with maternal cigarette smoking probably is largely dependent on reduced linear skeletal growth of the fetus, as has been demonstrated in the published studies that have investigated linear skeletal growth as well as birth weights of infants born to smoking and nonsmoking mothers.[5-7] The reduction in mean birth weight of 180 gm that has been calculated to occur in infants of

TABLE 11–2.—INCIDENCE OF
FULL-TERM SHORT-FOR-DATES
(SHFD*) INFANTS ACCORDING TO
NUMBER OF CIGARETTES SMOKED
PER DAY DURING PREGNANCY BY
GRAVIDAS

NUMBER OF CIGARETTES REPORTED SMOKED PER DAY	FULL-TERM INFANTS		
	Total	SHFD	
	No.	No.	%
≥ 21	123	23	18.7
11 – 20	268	46	17.1
6 – 10	137	20	14.6
1 – 5	61	5	8.2
0	1399	85	6.1

*SHFD (≤ fifth percentile, Tables 4-2 and 4-3).

mothers who smoke can be accounted for by the reduction in mean crown-heel length of 1 cm that has been observed in each of the studies cited.

The pathogenesis of the fetal growth retardation observed in newborn infants of mothers who smoked during pregnancy has not been finally settled. Among the 3000 chemical compounds that have been identified in inhaled cigarette smoke, nicotine and carbon monoxide have received the most attention. Longo[12] has reviewed the biologic effects of carbon monoxide in cigarette smoke on mothers, fetuses and newborn infants. The reports by the Surgeon General of the United States summarize studies relating to the possible effects of nicotine.[9, 10] Both nicotine and carbon monoxide have their strong adherents and experiments in animals lend support to either as a possible etiologic agent. The possibility that both nicotine and carbon monoxide can affect fetal growth should be considered along with other unexplored possibilities.

In this chapter, mothers were excluded, except as noted, if any of the growth-retarding factors in Table 3-1 were present other than cigarette smoking during pregnancy. The mothers were white and were delivered consecutively of single infants at The University of Kansas Medical Center.

The incidences of premature births are shown in Table 11-1 according to the number of cigarettes smoked per day by mothers throughout pregnancy. Information on the amount of cigarettes smoked per day was obtained by the senior author in a personal interview with each mother between her delivery and discharge from the Medical Center. Some concept of the number of cigarettes smoked per day by mothers was obtained by noting the presence and absence of cigarette packs, lighters and ashtrays at each mother's bedside and counting the number of cigarette butts present in the ashtrays. Some women reported that they did not smoke, but on further questioning revealed that they had stopped as soon as they learned they were pregnant, usually after several weeks or months of pregnancy. In Table 11-1 there was a direct and significant relationship between the number of cigarettes smoked per day and the incidence of premature births. The incidence rose from 2.4% among infants of nonsmokers to 8.2% among mothers smoking more than 20 cigarettes a day. The increase in incidence of premature births among mothers who smoked 1–5 cigarettes a day was 3.1% and was not significantly greater than the incidence of 2.4% among non-smokers.

In Table 11–2, the incidence of short-for-dates (SHFD) full-term infants increased significantly as the number of cigarettes smoked per day increased. Among nonsmokers, the incidence of SHFD infants was 6.1% and increased to 18.7% among infants of mothers smoking more than 20 cigarettes per day. The increase of SHFD infants among women smoking 1–5 cigarettes per day was 8.2% and was not significantly higher than the incidence of 6.1% among nonsmokers.

Some women smoked only during a part of pregnancy (Table 11–3). The number was small. There was some slight increase in births of SHFD full-term infants when smoking was reported to have been limited to the first trimester or the last two trimesters of pregnancy.

Cigarette smoking by mothers in this study was not associated with significant increases in births of full-term infants with low ponderal indices or small occipitofrontal circumferences.

Maternal cigarette smoking during pregnancy was the most frequently observed of all the growth-retarding factors listed in Table 3–1. Cigarette smoking was adopted during pregnancy by 40% of all white mothers delivered at The University of Kansas Medical Center. The incidence of mothers who smoked during pregnancy varied from 15% in the highest socioeconomic group

TABLE 11–3.—PREGNANCY OUTCOME
AMONG WOMEN WHO REPORTED
SMOKING MORE THAN 5 CIGARETTES A
DAY THROUGH A PART OF PREGNANCY

TRIMESTERS OF PREGNANCY	TOTAL	INFANTS PREMATURE (< 37 WEEKS)	SHFD°
	No.	No.	No.
Tri 1	35	0	3
Tri 1 + 2	9	0	0
Tri 2 + 3	22	1	2
Total	66	1	5

°SHFD, short-for-dates (≤ fifth percentile, Tables 4-2 and 4-3).

(professional and managerial personnel) to 60% among unemployed white women. Cigarette smoking was found in frequent combination with all other growth-retarding factors.

Data in this study suggest that there are at least three factors that may interfere with linear skeletal growth of fetuses — maternal cigarette smoking, short maternal stature and a low maternal weight gain in pregnancy. When cigarette smoking occurred in combination with either a short maternal stature or a low maternal weight gain in pregnancy, the incidences of short-for-dates (SHFD) infants were increased above the incidences observed when these three factors occurred singly (Table 11–4). The incidences of SHFD infants among mothers who had either a low weight gain or smoked cigarettes or were of short stature were 10.8%, 15.9% and 8.4%, respectively. The incidence of SHFD infants born to mothers who smoked and also had low weight gains was 20.8%, and for mothers who were of short stature and smoked cigarettes the incidence of SHFD infants was 31.7%.

A special effort was made to determine if cigarette smoking by women during pregnancy had a teratogenic effect on the fetus. The study included 1032 white mothers who had none of the growth-retarding factors in their pregnancies listed in Table 3–1 and 574 white mothers whose only known growth-retarding factor was that they smoked cigarettes during pregnancies. All 1606 infants were seen by the senior author at birth and all their moth-

TABLE 11–4.—INCIDENCES OF FULL-TERM
SHORT-FOR-DATES (SHFD) INFANTS BORN TO MOTHERS
WITH SINGLE AND COMBINED FETAL
GROWTH-RETARDING FACTORS

SINGLE FACTORS	FULL-TERM INFANTS			COMBINED FACTORS	FULL-TERM INFANTS		
	Total No.	SHFD§ No.	%		Total No.	SHFD§ No.	%
LWG°	111	12	10.8	LWG° and smoking†	119	25	20.8
Cigarette smoking†	589	94	15.9				
Short maternal stature‡	95	8	8.4	Short stature‡ and smoking†	41	13	31.7

°LWG, low weight gains (≤ 227 gm, 1/2 lb per week, trimesters 2 and 3).
†Cigarette smoking, 1 or more cigarettes a day throughout pregnancy.
‡Short maternal stature (≤ 155 cm, 61 in.).
§SHFD (≤ fifth percentile, Tables 4-2 and 4-3).

ers were interviewed by him. The mothers were delivered consecutively at The University of Kansas Medical Center. The hospital records of the 1606 infants, all of whom were born after 37 completed weeks of gestation, subsequently were reviewed by the senior author and Dr. Grace Holmes, Assistant Professor of Pediatrics, at The University of Kansas. The infants were liveborn between March, 1973, and September, 1976. Any infant with a recognizable congenital malformation among the group of 1606 infants was included in the study. Each infant was seen and examined thoroughly on admission and on discharge from the newborn nursery. All malformations diagnosed in the nursery were confirmed by specialists, including pediatric cardiologists, orthopedic surgeons, ophthalmologists, plastic surgeons and pediatric surgeons. There were 64 infants who had congenital malformations diagnosed in the newborn nursery. The incidence of infants with congenital malformations was 3.6% among the 1032 nonsmokers and 4.7% among 574 mothers who smoked; the difference was not statistically significant by the chi-square test. The incidence of infants with congenital malformations born to smoking mothers was not dose-related to the number of cigarettes smoked per day. Support for the hypothesis that cigarette smoking has a teratogenic effect on the fetus was not obtained in this study, which was not definitive. The study did not include prenatal deaths nor infants whose congenital malformations were unrecognized at birth but became manifest after discharge from the nursery.

TABLE 11-5.—INCIDENCES OF LOW BIRTH WEIGHT (LBW) INFANTS (< 2500 GM) ACCORDING TO NUMBER OF CIGARETTES SMOKED BY THEIR MOTHERS THROUGHOUT PREGNANCY

NUMBER OF CIGARETTES REPORTED SMOKED PER DAY	INFANTS					
		Premature		Full-term		
	Total births No.	LBW		Total No.	LBW	
		No.	%		No.	%
≥ 21	134	8	6.0	123	3	2.4
11-20	285	16	5.6	268	6	2.2
6-10	146	7	4.8	137	3	2.2
1-5	63	2	3.2	61	1	1.6
0	1434	21	1.5	1399	4	0.3

Low birth weight infants. — The incidences of LBW infants born according to the number of cigarettes smoked per day throughout pregnancy reported by their mothers are shown in Table 11–5. The incidence of LBW premature infants rose steadily and significantly from 1.5% among women who reported not smoking during pregnancy to 6.0% among mothers who smoked more than 20 cigarettes a day. There was a similar steady increase in births of LBW full-term infants from 0.3% among mothers reporting no smoking to 2.4% among mothers who reported smoking more than 20 cigarettes a day.

REFERENCES

1. Kline, J., Stein, Z. A., Susser, M., and Warburton, D.: Smoking: A risk factor for spontaneous abortion, N. Engl. J. Med. 297:793, 1977.
2. Meyer, M. D., and Tonascia, J. A.: Maternal smoking, pregnancy complications and perinatal mortality, Am. J. Obstet. Gynecol. 128: 494, 1977.
3. Simpson, W. J.: A preliminary report on cigarette smoking and the incidence of prematurity, Am. J. Obstet. Gynecol. 73:808, 1957.
4. Lowe, C. R.: Effect of mothers' smoking habits on birth weight of their children, Br. Med. J. 2:673, 1959.
5. Hardy, J. B., and Mellits, E. D.: Does maternal smoking during pregnancy have a long-term effect on the child?, Lancet 2:1332, 1972.
6. Kullander, S., and Kallen, B.: A prospective study of smoking and pregnancy, Acta Obstet. Gynecol. Scand. 50:83, 1971.
7. Miller, H. C., and Hassanein, K.: Maternal smoking and fetal growth of full-term infants, Pediatr. Res. 8:960, 1974.
8. Miller, H. C., Hassanein, K., and Hensleigh, P.: Effects of behavioral and medical variables on fetal growth retardation, Am. J. Obstet. Gynecol. 127:643, 1977.
9. United States Public Health Service: The Health Consequences of Smoking: A Report of the Surgeon General: 1971 (United States Government Printing Office, Washington, D. C., 1971).
10. United States Public Health Service: The Health Consequences of Smoking: A Report of the Surgeon General: 1972, 1973 (Government Printing Office, Washington, D. C., 1972 and 1973).
11. Rush, D.: Examination of the relationship between birth weight, cigarette smoking during pregnancy and maternal weight gain, J. Obstet. Gynaecol. Br. Commonw. 81:746, 1974.
12. Longo, L. D.: The biological effects of carbon monoxide on the pregnant woman, fetus and newborn infant, Am. J. Obstet. Gynecol. 129:69, 1977.

12 / Lack of Prenatal Care

LACK OF PRENATAL CARE has been viewed by obstetricians as poor for both mother and baby. In *Williams' Obstetrics,* Pritchard and MacDonald[1] urge that each gravida register for professional prenatal care as soon as pregnancy is suspected, so that abnormal signs and evidence of trouble can be identified as early as possible and treated accordingly. Data on pregnancy outcome for women receiving little or no prenatal care are few. In the Collaborative Perinatal Study sponsored by the National Institutes of Health, a decline in stillbirth and neonatal death rates was observed among both black and white women who registered for prenatal care late in pregnancy.[2] Mothers were accepted in the study only if they had at least one prenatal visit, thereby creating an artifact that would favor pregnancy outcome among women who registered late in pregnancy. Stillbirths and neonatal death rates that occurred among early registrants would be excluded from the group of women who registered late. In the present study based on white women delivered consecutively of single, live-born infants at The University of Kansas Medical Center, mothers were accepted into the study irrespective of whether or not they had any prenatal care. The main interest was centered on gravidas who had little or no prenatal care.

Pregnancy outcome was poor among the 120 women who had 0–3 prenatal visits. There were only 27 of the 120 women who had pregnancies that were judged to have been free from all other growth-retarding factors listed in Table 3–1. It can be seen from Table 12–1 that the incidence of premature births among the 120 mothers with 0–3 visits was high (17.5%) and that it was uniformly high irrespective of whether mothers had medical complications or behavioral conditions or no known growth-retarding factors in their pregnancies. The incidence of premature births was as high among mothers who had 3 prenatal visits as it was among mothers who had fewer visits. There was a notable

TABLE 12–1.–INCIDENCE OF PREMATURE BIRTHS (< 37 COMPLETED WEEKS OF GESTATION) ACCORDING TO NUMBER OF PRENATAL VISITS AND THE PRESENCE OF GROWTH-RETARDING FACTORS AMONG MOTHERS

NUMBER OF PRENATAL VISITS BY GRAVIDAS	NO. OF PREMATURE INFANTS BORN TO MOTHERS WITH A GROWTH-RETARDING FACTOR									
	None		Behavioral* conditions		Medical† complications		GRAND TOTAL			
	Infants		Infants		Infants				Premature	
	Total No.	Premature No.	Total No.	Premature No.	Total No.	Premature No.	Total No.	No.	%
0–3	27	4	76	15	17	2	120	21	17.5
4–8	29	1	52	1	10	2	91	4	4.4
9–12	29	0	26	0	12	0	67	0	0.0
Total	85	5(5.9%)	154	16(10.4%)	39	4(10.3%)	278	25	9.0

*Behavioral conditions listed in Table 3-1.
†Medical complications of pregnancy listed in Table 3-1.

TABLE 12-2.—INCIDENCES OF UNDERGROWN
FULL-TERM INFANTS ACCORDING TO NUMBER
OF PRENATAL VISITS BY MOTHERS WITH NO
KNOWN GROWTH-RETARDING FACTORS
IN THEIR PREGNANCIES

	FULL-TERM INFANTS		
NUMBER OF PRENATAL VISITS	Total No.	LPI° No.	SHFD† No.	Small OF‡ circ. No.
0-3	23	0	5	0
4-8	28	2	0	0
9-12	29	4	1	0
Total	80	6(7.5%)	6(7.5%)	0

°LPI, low ponderal index (< fifth percentile, Table 4-5).
†SHFD, short-for-dates (≤ fifth percentile, Tables 4-2 and 4-3).
‡Small OF, occipitofrontal circumferences (≤ fifth percentile, Tables 4-7 and 4-8).

drop in premature births among women who had 4-12 visits; the incidence was 4.4% among women who had 4-8 visits and zero among women who had 9-12 visits. The data in Table 12-1 show that 15 of 25 total premature infants were born to women with behavioral conditions in their pregnancies who had 0-3 visits.

Pregnancy outcome for full-term infants is shown in Table

TABLE 12-3.—INCIDENCES OF UNDERGROWN
FULL-TERM INFANTS ACCORDING TO NUMBER OF
PRENATAL VISITS MADE BY MOTHERS WITH
BEHAVIORAL CONDITIONS IN THEIR PREGNANCIES

	FULL-TERM INFANTS		
NUMBER OF PRENATAL VISITS	Total No.	LPI° No.	SHFD† No.	Small OF‡ circ. No.
0-3	61	7	10	1
4-8	51	4	13	5
9-12	26	4	7	1
Total	138	15(10.9%)	30(21.7%)	7(5.1%)

°LPI, low ponderal index (< fifth percentile, Table 4-5).
†SHFD, short-for-dates (≤ fifth percentile, Tables 4-2 and 4-3).
‡Small OF, occipitofrontal circumferences (≤ fifth percentile, Tables 4-7 and 4-8).

12–2 for women with no other known growth-retarding factors in their pregnancies and in Table 12–3 for women with one or more of the seven behavioral conditions listed in Table 3–1. In Table 12–2 there were 5 short-for-dates infants (21.7%) born to the 23 mothers with 0–3 visits who had no other known growth-retarding factors. In Table 12–3 there were 7 infants with low ponderal indices (11.5%) and 10 short-for-dates infants (16.4%) born to 61 mothers with 0–3 visits who had behavioral conditions in their pregnancies. Births of short-for-dates infants were also high among mothers with behavioral conditions who had 4–12 visits.

Low birth weight infants. – The incidence of LBW infants was high (19.2%) among the 120 mothers with 0–3 visits (Table 12–4). Most of the latter increase in births of LBW infants was related to the large number of premature births in this group of women (17.5%), as shown in Table 12–1. The incidence of LBW infants was 12.1% among 91 women with 4–8 visits and 3.0% among 67 women with 9–12 visits. The lower incidences of LBW infants in the latter two groups of women were related to lower incidences of premature births.

Difficulties were encountered in calculating the incidence of full-term infants who were short-for-dates or had small occipito-frontal circumferences and were born to mothers who had 0–3 visits. The diagnosis of these two parameters of fetal under-growth requires knowing the infants' gestational ages. Half the women who had 0–3 visits and gave birth to full-term infants either did not know or were unsure of their pregnancy dates. The data on undergrown full-term infants in Tables 12–2 and 12–3

TABLE 12–4. – INCIDENCE OF LOW BIRTH WEIGHT (LBW) INFANTS (< 2500 GM) ACCORDING TO NUMBER OF PRENATAL VISITS BY WHITE GRAVIDAS

| NUMBER OF PRENATAL VISITS | INFANTS | | | | | TOTAL LBW INFANTS | |
| | | Premature (< 37 weeks) | | Full-term infants | | | |
	Total No.	Total No.	LBW No.	Total No.	LBW No.	No.	%
0–3	120	21	19	99	4	23	19.2
4–8	91	4	4	87	7	11	12.1
9–12	67	0	0	67	2	2	3.0
Total	278	25	23	253	13	36	12.6

were based on the total number of full-term births and not on just those born to mothers with known dates. The incidences of SHFD infants and infants with small OF circumferences in the group of mothers with 0–3 visits might have been higher had more of these mothers been sure of their pregnancy dates. Pregnancy dates were much better known among women who had 4–12 visits; about 90% of these women were sure of their dates and their calculated and estimated dates were in agreement.

It is difficult even to speculate as to why women with no other known growth-retarding factors who had fewer than 4 prenatal visits had increased births of premature infants and of full-term infants who were short-for-dates. The number of women who had 0–3 visits and were judged to have been free from known growth-retarding factors, as listed in Table 3–1, was small (27) and possibly larger numbers of them might have produced lower incidences of premature births and of short-for-dates infants. In general, the 27 control mothers who had 0–3 visits were younger and more likely to have been single, had fewer years of formal education and had a poorer socioeconomic status than women with 4–12 visits; 11 of the 27 control mothers with 0–3 visits were classified in the nonpoverty group and 16 in the poverty group, as defined in Chapter 5. The 4 premature infants born in the group of 27 mothers were equally divided between the nonpoverty and poverty groups. The possibility exists that the incidence of premature births would have been high even had the mothers with 0–3 visits begun their prenatal visits earlier and had more visits. Most of the 21 premature births in the group of 120 women with 0–3 visits followed a spontaneous onset of labor; 5 of the 21 births followed artificial induction of labor because of a premature, spontaneous rupture of membranes. More study should be undertaken to look for unknown and as yet unrecognized factors that might account for the poor pregnancy outcome among women with little or no prenatal care.

REFERENCES

1. Pritchard, J. A., and MacDonald, P. C.: *Williams' Obstetrics* (15th ed.; New York: Appleton-Century-Crofts, 1976).
2. The Collaborative Perinatal Study of the National Institutes of Neurological Disease and Stroke: The Women and Their Pregnancies. Department of Health, Education, and Welfare Publication No. (NIH) 73-379, Washington, D. C., U. S. Department of Health, Education, and Welfare, 1972.

13 / Addicting Drugs and Chronic Alcoholism

THERE WERE FEW WHITE MOTHERS delivered at The University of Kansas Medical Center who were chronic alcoholics or used addicting drugs. This low incidence was not related to inadequate diagnosis but to the comparatively low incidence of gravidas in the general population of white mothers in the area who use addicting drugs or are chronic alcoholics. In the period of 5 years covered by this study of fetal growth in offspring of white women delivered at this Medical Center, 10 mothers were identified as taking methadone during pregnancy, 3 of them also being on heroin occasionally; 6 mothers were diagnosed as chronic alcoholics.

It is worthwhile considering these mothers as a single group from the viewpoint of their behavior during pregnancy. All 16 mothers were involved with other behavioral conditions besides being on addicting drugs or being chronic alcoholics; 14 mothers reported smoking cigarettes heavily during pregnancy, averaging more than 30 cigarettes a day (range 10–60); 8 mothers had low weight gains during pregnancy (≤ 227 gm, ½ lb, per week in the last two trimesters); 4 were underweight at conception; 2 had no prenatal care; 2 were less than 17 years of age at delivery. Two mothers had four behavioral conditions each; 8 mothers had three behavioral conditions and the remaining 6 mothers had two each. Two mothers had blood hemoglobin levels of less than 8.5 gm/dl; 1 mother had hepatitis during her pregnancy; there were no other medical complications identified in these 16 women. Their poor pregnancy outcome reflected their status during pregnancy; 6 mothers had early onset of spontaneous labor before 37 weeks of completed pregnancy and 5 of their 6 infants had birth weights under 2500 gm; 6 other infants were born after 37 weeks and were short-for-dates (crown-heel lengths

$\leq$ fifth percentile, Tables 4–2 and 4–3); 2 infants had small occipitofrontal circumferences ($\leq$ fifth percentile, Tables 4–7 and 4–8); 1 infant had a low ponderal index (< fifth percentile, Table 4–5); there were 2 of the 16 infants who were not undergrown in some way and were not born prematurely.

Methadone. — The 10 mothers on methadone were in a special treatment program. Their dosage of methadone ranged from 12 to 45 mg a day. All 10 mothers smoked cigarettes during pregnancy; 4 of the 10 mothers also had low weight gains during pregnancy. One mother was anemic (hgb, 8.4 gm/dl); the other 9 mothers had none of the medical complications of pregnancy listed in Table 3–1. Nine of the 10 infants either were born prematurely or were severely undergrown if they were full-term. The most frequently observed evidence of undergrowth was a short crown-heel length for the full-term infant's gestational age; 5 of the 10 infants were short-for-dates and 1 of the 5 infants also had a small occipitofrontal circumference for his gestational age. A sixth infant had a small occipitofrontal circumference. A seventh infant was severely malnourished and had a ponderal index of 2.15, well below the fifth percentile (see Table 4–5). Two infants were born prematurely. There was only 1 of the 10 infants who appeared to have normal fetal growth; the mother was on the lowest dose of methadone (12 mg per day) in the group of 10 mothers. It was impossible in this group of 10 white infants to attribute their poor pregnancy outcome to methadone or any one other single factor, especially because all 10 mothers were heavy cigarette smokers during pregnancy and 4 mothers also had low weight gains during pregnancy. Previous investigators have suggested that multiple factors may be involved in the reduction of birth weights of infants born to mothers on addicting drugs, but they have not documented or evaluated all the additional potential growth-retarding factors.[1, 2]

Alcohol. — Six mothers were considered by the Obstetric Service to be heavy consumers of alcohol and chronic alcoholics throughout pregnancy. Each of the 6 mothers had from one to three additional behavioral conditions; 4 were heavy cigarette smokers during pregnancy; 3 were underweight at conception; 2 women had low weight gains in their pregnancies; 1 mother was over 35 years of age and 1 was 16 years of age. One mother had hepatitis during her pregnancy. None of the other 5 mothers had any of the medical complications of pregnancy listed in Table 3–1. Pregnancy outcome was poor for the 6 infants; 4 were born prematurely after premature spontaneous onset of labors and had birth weights ranging from 1200 to 1950 gm. One full-term infant was short-for-dates; the other full-term infant had no evidence of fetal undergrowth. None of the 6 infants was identified as having the fetal alcohol syndrome. The reason for including these 6 mothers and infants was mainly to illustrate that mothers who consume large amounts of alcohol during pregnancy are likely to be involved with other behavioral conditions that may affect fetal growth. One of the cardinal features of the fetal alcohol syndrome is a reduction in skeletal length.[3, 4] We have shown that both cigarette smoking and low weight gains during pregnancy may be associated with significant reductions in fetal skeletal length; these two factors should be taken into account in evaluating fetal growth of infants of alcoholic mothers.

REFERENCES

1. Blinick, G., Wallach, R. C., Jerez, E., and Ackerman, B. D.: Drug addiction in pregnancy and the neonate, Am. J. Obstet. Gynecol. 125: 135, 1976.
2. Kandall, S. R., Albin, S., Lowinson, J., Berle, B., Eidelman, A. I., and Gartner, L. M.: Differential effects of maternal heroin and methadone use on birth weight, Pediatrics 58:681, 1976.
3. Hanson, J. W., Jones, K. L., and Smith, D. W.: Fetal alcohol syndrome: Experience with 41 patients, JAMA 235:1458, 1976.
4. Ouellette, E. M., Rosett, H. L., Rosman, N. P., and Weinder, L.: Adverse effects of maternal alcohol abuse during pregnancy, N. Engl. J. Med. 297:528, 1977.

14 / Complications of Pregnancy

INVESTIGATORS have recognized for a long time that certain maternal complications during pregnancy of an organic nature have been associated with an increased incidence of premature births and with fetal growth retardation. Data are presented in this chapter that support the results obtained by previous investigators.

There were 435 white mothers who had either medical or obstetric complications in their pregnancies and were delivered of single infants at The University of Kansas Medical Center. Their complications were of the types listed under group II, Table 3–1. The diagnoses of their complications were obtained from their medical and obstetric hospital records; 421 mothers had a single complication and 14 had two complications. The latter 14 mothers will not be considered further. The 421 mothers with single complications were separated into two groups; one group had complications of an obstetric nature and the other group had complications that were more medical than obstetric. Each of these two groups was subdivided into two groups; one group had complications only and the other group of mothers had complications and also one or more of the seven behavioral conditions listed in Table 3–1.

There were 152 mothers who had complications that were more medical than obstetric; 87 of the 152 mothers had a single complication and also one or more behavioral conditions; the remaining 65 mothers had a single medical complication and none of the other growth-retarding factors in Table 3–1. Pregnancy outcome in the latter group of 65 mothers is shown in Table 14–1. The number of mothers with similar medical problems was too small to provide a satisfactory statistical analysis for any one problem. It is clear, however, that in the combined group of 65 women, the incidences of premature births and of undergrown full-term infants were unusually high. There were 6 pre-

TABLE 14–1.–PREGNANCY OUTCOME AMONG WOMEN WITH A SINGLE MEDICAL COMPLICATION IN PREGNANCY AND NO OTHER GROWTH-RETARDING FACTORS

MEDICAL COMPLICATIONS	TOTAL BIRTHS NO.	PREMATURE INFANTS (< 37 wk) TOTAL NO.	FULL-TERM INFANTS			
			Total No.	LPI* No.	SHFD† No.	Small OF‡ No.
Neuropsychiatric	9	0	9	2	1	1
Chronic hypertension	8	1	7	0	1	0
Asthma	8	1	7	1	1	0
Epilepsy	8	0	8	2	1	1
Ulcerative colitis	5	1	4	1	0	1
Thyroid disease	7	0	7	1	1	1
Renal disease	5	2	3	0	2	2
Cancers	3	0	3	1	1	0
Anemia (hgb < 10 gm/dl)	3	1	2	0	1	0
Rh hemolytic disease	2	0	2	0	1	0
Liver disease	1	0	1	1	0	0
Rheumatoid arthritis	1	0	1	1	0	0
Mitral insufficiency (compensated)	1	0	1	1	0	0
Aspergillosis	1	0	1	0	0	0
Pyelonephritis (recurrent)	1	0	1	0	0	0
Quadraplegia	1	0	1	0	0	0
Indural medication	1	0	1	0	1	0
Total	65	6(9.2%)	59	11(18.6%)	11(18.6%)	6(10%)

*LPI, low ponderal index (< fifth percentile, Table 4-5).
†SHFD, short-for-dates (≤ fifth percentile, Tables 4-2 and 4-3).
‡Small OF, occipitofrontal circumferences (≤ fifth percentile, Tables 4-7 and 4-8).

mature births (9.2%), 5 of which resulted from premature, spontaneous onsets of labor. Among the 59 full-term infants, 11 (18.6%) had low ponderal indices and 11 (18.6%) were short-for-dates. Small occipitofrontal circumferences were observed in 6 infants (10%). Many of the 65 mothers were taking drugs for their medical problems. It was not possible to determine how much the drugs contributed to an unsatisfactory pregnancy outcome. Pregnancy outcome among the 87 mothers who had behavioral conditions in addition to their medical complications was not significantly different from pregnancy outcome in the group of 65 mothers with no behavioral conditions. The similarity of pregnancy outcome among mothers who had medical complications with and without behavioral conditions suggests that their medical problems were the overriding factors in their poor pregnancy outcome.

There were 269 mothers who had obstetric problems during pregnancy; 145 of the 269 mothers had one obstetric problem each and no other fetal growth-retarding factors in their pregnancies of the types listed in Table 3–1. The incidence of premature births was high (Table 14–2); 21 premature infants (14.5%) were born in the group of 145 mothers and 10 of the 21 premature births followed labors that were artificially induced because of the obstetric problems. There was a high incidence of full-term infants who had low ponderal indices; 14 (11.3%) of 124 full-term infants had low ponderal indices. The incidence of full-term short-for-dates infants was 7.3%, which is slightly higher than the expected rate of 5% (the diagnosis of SHFD is based on a crown-heel length at or below the fifth percentile for fetal age). The over-all incidence of full-term infants with small occipitofrontal circumferences was 4.1% and not significantly different from the expected rate of 5%. The mothers who had acute hypertension (blood pressure $\geq$ 130/80 mm Hg) were hypertensive at or near delivery and had no proteinuria, headaches, blurring of vision or hyperactive reflexes. Vaginal bleeding was associated with placenta previas, marginal sinus rupture, abruptio placentae or was of uncertain etiology. Abnormal placentas included battledore, bilobed, bipartite, succenturiate and circumvallate placentas and placenta accreta.

The combination of obstetric complications and behavioral conditions in 124 mothers in Table 14–3 was associated with

TABLE 14–2.—PREGNANCY OUTCOME AMONG MOTHERS WITH OBSTETRIC COMPLICATIONS OF PREGNANCY BUT NO OTHER KNOWN GROWTH-RETARDING FACTORS

OBSTETRIC COMPLICATIONS OF PREGNANCY	TOTAL INFANTS NO.	PREMATURE INFANTS (< 37 WK) TOTAL NO.	FULL-TERM INFANTS			
			Total No.	LPI° No.	SHFD† No.	Small OF‡ circ. No.
Preeclampsia	85	14	71	7	4	2
Acute hypertension	25	0	25	3	3	1
Vaginal bleeding (third trimester)	22	3	19	2	1	2
Abnormal placenta	9	2	7	1	1	0
Abnormal uterus	2	2	0	0	0	0
Hydramnios	2	0	2	1	0	0
Total	145	21(14.5%)	124	14(11.3%)	9(7.3%)	5(4.1%)

°, † and ‡ same as in Table 14-1.

TABLE 14-3.—COMPARISON OF PREGNANCY OUTCOME AMONG MOTHERS WITH
OBSTETRIC COMPLICATIONS ACCORDING TO PRESENCE OR ABSENCE
OF BEHAVIORAL CONDITIONS§

MOTHERS WITH OBSTETRIC COMPLICATIONS	NO.	PREMATURE INFANTS (< 37 WK)		Total births No.	FULL-TERM INFANTS					
		NO.	%		LPI*		SHFD†		Small OF‡ circ.	
					No.	%	No.	%	No.	%
No behavioral conditions	145	21	14.5	124	14	11.3	9	7.3	5	4.1
Behavioral conditions	124	28	22.6	96	9	9.4	18	18.4	14	14.6

*, †, and ‡ same as in Table 14-1.
§Behavioral conditions as listed under group III, Table 3-1.

increased births of premature infants and of full-term infants who were short-for-dates or had small occipitofrontal circumferences. The incidence of premature births among the 124 mothers was 22.6% and among 145 mothers with obstetric complications and no behavioral conditions it was 14.5%. The incidence of full-term infants who were short-for-dates among mothers who had obstetric complications and behavioral conditions was 18.4% and more than twice that among mothers with obstetric complications and no behavioral conditions. Infants with small OF circumferences occurred 3 times more frequently among mothers with behavioral conditions shown in Table 14-3 than among mothers without behavioral conditions.

Low birth weight infants. — There were 82 infants (19.4%) with birth weights under 2500 gm born to 421 mothers with single medical or obstetric complications of pregnancy. The incidence was lower among 210 mothers who had no behavioral conditions (16.2%) than among 211 mothers with behavioral conditions (22.7%).

15 / Black Mothers and Their Infants

DATA IN THIS CHAPTER are based on 1210 black mothers delivered of single infants consecutively at The University of Kansas Medical Center as part of the over-all study on fetal growth. Most of the mothers had either behavioral conditions or medical complications in their pregnancies, leaving less than half who had no known growth-retarding factors of the types listed in Table 3–1. Some of the latter mothers were uncertain about the dates of their last menstrual periods, leaving 473 mothers and their full-term infants who fit our criteria for purposes of constructing standards of fetal growth (Tables 15–1 to 15–6). Black infants were selected as controls, using the same criteria as used for white infants in Chapter 4. Also, the data on crown-heel lengths, head circumferences and birth weights in Tables 15–1 to 15–6 were prepared in the same way as were data in the tables for standards for white infants in Chapter 4. The 473 infants were about equally divided between boys and girls and between those born to primiparas and multiparas.

Crown-heel length. – The distribution of crown-heel lengths of full-term black control infants is shown for boys in Table 15–1 and for girls in Table 15–2. Black control infants tended to be shorter than white control infants of the same gestational ages. The crown-heel lengths of black control infants were affected by the same factors as were observed in white control infants, including gestational age, sex, maternal height and to a slight extent by parity (primipara versus multipara). In both boys and girls, those born to primiparas had mean crown-heel lengths that were about 0.3 mm shorter than boys and girls of the same gestational age born to multiparas. Infants born to primiparas and multiparas, however, were combined in Tables 15–1 and 15–2, because the total number of control infants was relatively small

TABLE 15-1.—DISTRIBUTION OF CROWN-HEEL LENGTHS (CM) OF BLACK NEWBORN MALE INFANTS (CONTROLS) BY PERCENTILES ACCORDING TO THEIR GESTATIONAL AGES

PERCENTILES	GESTATIONAL AGES—WEEKS					
	37	38	39	40	41	42-43
95	51.5	52.5	53.5	54.5	54.5	54.5
90	51.0	52.0	52.7	53.5	54.0	54.0
75	50.5	51.5	52.0	52.5	53.0	53.0
50	49.5	50.0	50.5	51.0	51.5	52.0
25	48.5	49.0	49.5	50.0	50.5	51.0
10	47.5	48.0	48.5	49.0	49.5	50.0
5	47.0	47.5	48.0	48.5	49.0	49.5

TABLE 15-2.—DISTRIBUTION OF CROWN-HEEL LENGTHS (CM) OF BLACK NEWBORN FEMALE INFANTS (CONTROLS) BY PERCENTILES ACCORDING TO THEIR GESTATIONAL AGES

PERCENTILES	GESTATIONAL AGE—WEEKS					
	37	38	39	40	41	42-43
95	51.0	51.7	52.5	53.3	54.0	54.0
90	50.3	51.0	51.8	52.5	53.5	53.0
75	49.5	50.5	51.0	51.5	52.0	52.5
50	49.0	49.5	50.0	50.5	51.0	51.5
25	48.0	48.5	49.0	49.5	50.0	50.5
10	47.0	47.5	48.0	48.5	49.0	49.5
5	46.5	47.0	47.5	48.0	48.5	49.0

TABLE 15-3.—DISTRIBUTION OF OCCIPITOFRONTAL CIRCUMFERENCES (CM) OF BLACK MALE INFANTS (CONTROLS) BY PERCENTILES ACCORDING TO THEIR GESTATIONAL AGES

PERCENTILES	GESTATIONAL AGE—WEEKS					
	37	38	39	40	41	42-43
95	35.3	35.8	36.2	36.7	37.0	37.0
90	35.0	35.5	35.9	36.3	36.7	36.8
75	34.6	34.9	35.3	35.6	36.0	36.3
50	33.6	34.0	34.4	34.7	35.1	35.5
25	33.1	33.4	33.8	34.1	34.5	34.9
10	32.4	32.8	33.1	33.4	33.8	34.1
5	32.1	32.5	32.8	33.1	33.4	33.7

in each gestational age group. Boys and girls born to control tall mothers had longer crown-heel lengths at birth than boys and girls of similar gestational age born to control short mothers.

Head size.—The distribution of occipitofrontal circumferences of full-term black control infants is shown for boys in Table 15–3 and for girls in Table 15–4 according to their gestational ages. Their head circumferences were affected by gestational age and sex but were not significantly affected by parity, height or prepregnancy habitus of their mothers. When sex and gestational ages of the infants were held constant, maternal prepregnancy habitus (weight-height ratio) did not significantly affect head circumference. When gestational ages, sex and maternal prepregnancy habitus were held constant, maternal height had no significant effect on occipitofrontal circumferences. In Table 7–4, a tenfold increase in incidence of infants with small occipitofrontal circumferences was noted among white control mothers who were underweight for their heights at conception, as compared to the incidence among obese white mothers. A similar trend was observed among black control mothers; the incidence of infants with small occipitofrontal circumferences (≤ fifth percentile for gestational age and sex) was 5.6% among infants of 178 black mothers whose prepregnancy habitus was above average (weight ≥ 7.5% above normal for height in Sargent's table[1]) and was 10.4% among 77 infants of black mothers whose prepregnancy habitus was below average (weight ≥ 7.5% below normal for height in Sargent's table). The difference between these two incidences was not statistically significant by the chi-square test.

TABLE 15–4.—DISTRIBUTION OF OCCIPITOFRONTAL CIRCUMFERENCES (CM) OF BLACK FEMALE INFANTS (CONTROLS) BY PERCENTILES ACCORDING TO THEIR GESTATIONAL AGES

PERCENTILES	GESTATIONAL AGE — WEEKS					
	37	38	39	40	41	42–43
95	35.0	35.1	35.6	35.9	36.2	36.5
90	34.3	34.8	35.3	35.6	35.8	36.0
75	34.1	34.3	34.6	34.8	35.1	35.3
50	33.4	33.6	33.9	34.1	34.4	34.7
25	32.7	33.0	33.2	33.5	33.7	34.0
10	32.1	32.3	32.6	32.8	33.1	33.3
5	31.7	32.0	32.2	32.5	32.8	33.0

TABLE 15–5.–DISTRIBUTION OF BIRTH WEIGHTS (KG) OF
BLACK NEWBORN MALE INFANTS (CONTROLS) BY
PERCENTILES ACCORDING TO THEIR
GESTATIONAL AGES

| PERCENTILES | GESTATIONAL AGE – WEEKS | | | | | |
	37	38	39	40	41	42–43
95	3.44	3.71	3.97	4.13	4.29	4.40
90	3.38	3.62	3.84	3.97	4.10	4.15
75	3.30	3.46	3.62	3.72	3.82	3.92
50	3.08	3.18	3.30	3.40	3.50	3.60
25	2.83	2.93	3.03	3.13	3.22	3.32
10	2.63	2.73	2.82	2.90	2.99	3.08
5	2.54	2.68	2.72	2.82	2.95	3.00

Birth weight.–The distribution of birth weights for full-term
black control infants is shown for boys in Table 15–5 and for
girls in Table 15–6 according to their gestational ages. Birth
weights of black control infants were affected by gestational age
and sex of the infants and by the parity, height and prepregnancy
habitus of their mothers. Separate tables were not prepared to
demonstrate the effects of maternal parity, height and prepregnancy
habitus because there were so few infants in each category.

Ponderal index.–In a previous study made at The University
of Kansas Medical Center, the ponderal indices of black full-
term control infants, using Rohrer's formula, were found to have
a distribution similar to that of white infants and to be affected by
parity but not by gestational age or sex.[2] It is our practice to use

TABLE 15–6.–DISTRIBUTION OF BIRTH WEIGHTS (KG) OF
BLACK NEWBORN FEMALE INFANTS (CONTROLS) BY
PERCENTILES ACCORDING TO THEIR
GESTATIONAL AGES

| PERCENTILES | GESTATIONAL AGE – WEEKS | | | | | |
	37	38	39	40	41	42–43
95	3.44	3.65	3.83	3.97	4.00	4.15
90	3.32	3.53	3.73	3.88	3.98	4.05
75	3.14	3.32	3.48	3.60	3.73	3.85
50	2.93	3.07	3.22	3.34	3.46	3.58
25	2.70	2.83	2.95	3.08	3.03	3.32
10	2.53	2.65	2.77	2.89	3.01	3.10
5	2.43	2.54	2.65	2.77	2.89	3.01

the distribution of ponderal indices shown in Table 4–5 for white control infants born to multipara in determining the percentiles for black infants.

Premature infants.—There were 109 premature infants (< 37 completed weeks of gestation) born to the group of 1210 black mothers, an incidence of 9%; 25 (23%) of the 109 premature infants were born to mothers with no known growth-retarding factors in their pregnancies of the types listed in Table 3–1. Many of the 109 mothers delivered of premature infants were uncertain about their menstrual dates. Premature infants whose calculated and estimated gestational ages were judged to be in agreement had birth weights not strikingly different from those observed in white premature infants shown in Figures 4–12 and 4–14. There were some differences in the birth weights of premature black infants born to control mothers and those born to mothers with medical complications and behavioral conditions in their pregnancies, just as there were among white premature infants, but the differences were not so marked among the black premature infants, possibly because there were fewer black mothers who smoked cigarettes heavily (> 20 cigarettes per day) during pregnancy.

The similarities and differences in pregnancy outcome between black mothers and white mothers are presented in the following pages.

With respect to socioeconomic status and growth-retarding factors, pregnancy outcome for black mothers generally followed the same trends as we observed among white mothers. The incidences of single, low birth weight (LBW) black infants born consecutively at The University of Kansas Medical Center were not significantly different among black mothers in the nonpoverty and poverty groups (Table 15–7). Criteria for classifying black mothers in nonpoverty and poverty groups were the same as those used for white mothers in Chapter 5. Further subdivision of black mothers into four socioeconomic groups was not carried out as it was for white mothers because there were too few black mothers in groups I and III. The few black mothers in groups I and III were combined with mothers in groups II and IV, respectively.

The lowest incidences of LBW black infants were among mothers who had no known growth-retarding factors in their

TABLE 15-7.—INCIDENCE OF LOW BIRTH WEIGHT BLACK INFANTS ACCORDING TO SOCIOECONOMIC STATUS AND PRESENCE OF GROWTH-RETARDING FACTORS IN MOTHERS

GROWTH-RETARDING FACTORS IN MOTHERS	NONPOVERTY					POVERTY				
		Infants					Infants			
	Total No.	< 2500 gm No.	%	< 2350 gm No.	%	Total No.	< 2500 gm No.	%	< 2350 gm No.	%
Medical complications*	65	21	32.3	18	27.7	87	19	21.8	16	22.1
Behavioral conditions†	197	27	13.7	20	10.1	339	51	15.0	31	9.1
None present‡	274	17	6.2	10	3.6	248	12	4.8	8	3.2

*Medical complications as listed under group II, Table 3-1.
†Behavioral conditions as listed under group III, Table 3-1.
‡None of the growth-retarding factors listed in Table 3-1.

pregnancies (see Table 15–7). Among the latter mothers, the incidence of LBW infants was about 3.5% and was increased to about 9.5% among mothers with behavioral conditions and to about 25% among mothers with medical complications in their pregnancies. The 536 black mothers in Table 15–7 who had one or more of the seven behavioral conditions listed in Table 3–1 and no other known growth-retarding factors in their pregnancies constituted the largest group of mothers and produced the largest number of LBW infants. There were no significant differences in the incidences of LBW infants < 2500 gm or of LBW infants < 2350 gm between the nonpoverty and poverty groups when mothers were separated according to whether they had medical complications or behavioral conditions or neither in their pregnancies. It is apparent that the poverty group had more mothers with behavioral problems and fewer control mothers than the nonpoverty group. A similar distribution was noted among white mothers in Chapter 5. The incidences of black mothers with medical complications in Table 15–7 were not significantly different between the nonpoverty and poverty groups.

The incidences of premature infants (< 37 completed weeks of gestation) are shown in Table 15–8 according to socioeconomic status and according to presence of growth-retarding factors in black mothers. The incidence of premature births was lowest among mothers with no known growth-retarding factors in their

TABLE 15–8.–INCIDENCE OF PREMATURE BLACK INFANTS (< 37 COMPLETED WEEKS OF GESTATION) ACCORDING TO SOCIOECONOMIC STATUS AND PRESENCE OF GROWTH-RETARDING FACTORS IN MOTHERS

| GROWTH-RETARDING FACTORS IN MOTHERS | NONPOVERTY | | | POVERTY | | |
| | Infants | | | Infants | | |
	Total No.	< 37 weeks No.	%	Total No.	< 37 weeks No.	%
Medical complications°	65	14	21.5	87	14	16.0
Behavioral conditions†	197	19	9.6	339	37	10.9
None present‡	274	18	6.6	248	7	2.8

°Medical complications as listed under group II, Table 3-1.
†Behavioral conditions as listed under group III, Table 3-1.
‡None of the growth-retarding factors listed in Table 3-1.

pregnancies and highest among mothers with medical complications. The incidences of premature births were not significantly higher among mothers in the poverty than among mothers in the nonpoverty groups. It is interesting to observe that the incidence of premature births among mothers with no known growth-retarding factors was significantly lower in the poverty than in the nonpoverty group (p < 0.05) by the chi-square test; one-third of the premature infants in the latter group were born following induction of labor for premature spontaneous rupture of membranes. More than half of the premature infants in Table 15–8 were born to mothers with behavioral conditions and the largest number were in the poverty group, containing as it did the larger number of mothers with behavioral conditions.

The incidences of severely undergrown full-term black infants are shown in Table 15–9 according to presence of growth-retarding factors in their mothers. The group of 124 mothers with medical complications in their pregnancies had 3 times as many infants with low ponderal indices as did the group of 497 control mothers. The group of 480 mothers with behavioral conditions had 65 infants (13.5%) who were short-for-dates; this incidence was statistically significantly higher than that of 7.2% in the control group of 497 mothers by the chi-square test, p < 0.05.

Cigarette smoking and low weight gains by mothers during pregnancy were the two most frequently observed behavioral

TABLE 15–9.—INCIDENCE OF FULL-TERM BLACK INFANTS WHO HAD LOW PONDERAL INDICES (LPI) OR WERE SHORT-FOR-DATES (SHFD) ACCORDING TO PRESENCE OF GROWTH-RETARDING FACTORS IN THEIR MOTHERS' PREGNANCIES

GROWTH-RETARDING FACTORS IN MOTHERS	FULL-TERM INFANTS				
	Total	LPI§		SHFD‖	
	No.	No.	%	No.	%
Medical complications°	124	19	15.3	14	11.3
Behavioral conditions†	480	33	6.9	65	13.5
None present‡	497	24	4.8	36	7.2

°Medical complications as listed under group II, Table 3-1.
†Behavioral conditions as listed under group III, Table 3-1.
‡None of the growth-retarding factors listed in Table 3-1.
§LPI (< fifth percentile, Table 4-5).
‖SHFD (≤ fifth percentile, Tables 15-1 and 15-2).

TABLE 15–10.—PREGNANCY OUTCOME AMONG BLACK MOTHERS WHO SMOKED CIGARETTES DURING PREGNANCY

BEHAVIORAL CONDITIONS IN MOTHERS	INFANTS			FULL-TERM INFANTS					
	Total No.	< 37 weeks* No.	%	Total No.	LPI† No.	%	SHFD‡ No.	%
Smokers only	227	23	10.1	204	9	4.4	35	17.1
Smokers and other behavioral conditions§	123	13	10.6	110	7	6.4	24	21.8
Total smokers	350	36	10.3	314	16	5.1	59	18.8
None present (controls)	522	25	4.8	497	24	4.8	36	7.2

*Under 37 completed weeks of gestation.
†LPI, low ponderal index (< fifth percentile, Table 4-5).
‡SHFD, short-for-dates (≤ fifth percentile, Tables 15-1 and 15-2).
§Other behavioral conditions include those under group III, Table 3-1.

conditions among black mothers, as was the case with white mothers. Pregnancy outcome among black mothers who smoked any amount of cigarettes during any part of pregnancy is shown in Table 15–10. The incidence of premature infants among 227 mothers whose only known growth-retarding factor in their pregnancies was cigarette smoking was 10.1% and was significantly higher than the incidence of premature infants among 522 control mothers by the chi-square test, p < 0.02. Also, the incidence of premature births among 123 mothers who smoked cigarettes and had one or more other behavioral conditions was 10.6% and was significantly higher than the incidence among control mothers, p < 0.01. There were no significant increases in births of full-term infants with low ponderal indices among mothers who smoked cigarettes during pregnancy. Births of short-for-dates full-term infants were significantly increased among mothers who smoked cigarettes as compared to births of SHFD infants among control mothers, p < 0.001.

There was a significant association between the amount of cigarette smoking by black mothers and the incidence of severe fetal growth retardation observed in full-term infants (Table 15–11). The mothers in Table 15–11 reported smoking throughout their pregnancies. They were not known to have any of the other growth-retarding factors in their pregnancies listed in Table 3–1. Black mothers who reported smoking 1–5 cigarettes a day had no significantly higher incidences of growth-retarded full-term infants than observed among controls. Mothers reporting that they smoked 6 or more cigarettes a day had significantly higher incidences of short-for-dates infants and infants with small occipitofrontal circumferences than mothers who reported no cigarette smoking, p being < 0.02 in each instance.

Pregnancy outcome among mothers with low weight gains (LWG) in pregnancy is shown in Table 15–12. The incidence of

TABLE 15–11.—INCIDENCE OF UNDERGROWN FULL-TERM
BLACK INFANTS ACCORDING TO NUMBER OF
CIGARETTES SMOKED PER DAY BY THEIR MOTHERS

NUMBER OF CIGARETTES SMOKED PER DAY	FULL-TERM INFANTS						
	Total No.	LPI°		SHFD†		Small OF‡ circ.	
		No.	%	No.	%	No.	%
> 10	47	2	4.3	13	27.7	7	14.9
6–10	66	3	4.6	12	18.2	6	9.1
1–5	42	2	4.8	3	7.1	3	7.1
0	497	24	4.8	36	7.2	26	5.2

°LPI, low ponderal index (< fifth percentile, Table 4-5).
†SHFD, short-for-dates (≤ fifth percentile, Tables 15-1 and 15-2).
‡OF, occipitofrontal (≤ fifth percentile, Tables 15-3 and 15-4).

TABLE 15–12.—PREGNANCY OUTCOME AMONG BLACK MOTHERS WITH LOW WEIGHT GAINS (LWG)* IN THEIR PREGNANCIES

BEHAVIORAL CONDITIONS IN MOTHERS	INFANTS			FULL-TERM INFANTS				
	Total No.	< 37 weeks† No.	%	Total No.	LPI‡ No.	%	SHFD§ No.	%
LWG only	70	3	4.3	67	9	13.4	6	9.0
LWG and other behavioral conditions‖	72	9	12.5	63	8	12.7	14	22.1
Total	142	12	8.4	130	17	13.1	20	15.4
None present (controls)	522	25	4.8	497	24	4.8	36	7.2

*LWG (≤ 227 gm per week in second and third trimesters).
†Under 37 completed weeks of gestation.
‡LPI, low ponderal index (< fifth percentile, Table 4-5).
§SHFD, short-for-dates (≤ fifth percentile, Tables 15-1 and 15-2).
‖Other behavioral conditions include those under group III, Table 3-1.

premature births among mothers who had LWG as their only known growth-retarding factor in their pregnancies was not significantly increased over the incidence among control mothers, but it was among mothers who had LWG and one or more of the other six behavioral conditions shown in Table 3–1. The differ-

TABLE 15–13.—PREGNANCY OUTCOME AMONG BLACK MOTHERS UNDERWEIGHT FOR HEIGHT AT CONCEPTION

	INFANTS			FULL-TERM INFANTS							
	Total No.	< 37 weeks No.	%	Total No.	LPI* No.	%	SHFD† No.	%	Small OF‡ circ. No.	%
Underweight§	69	12	17.4	57	7	12.3	10	17.5	5	8.8
Controls‖	522	25	4.8	497	24	4.8	36	7.2	26	5.2

*LPI, low ponderal index (< fifth percentile, Table 4-5).
†SHFD, short-for-dates (≤ fifth percentile, Tables 15-1 and 15-2).
‡Small OF, occipitofrontal circumferences (≤ fifth percentile, Tables 15-3 and 15-4).
§Weight was ≥ 15% below normal for height on Sargent's table.[1]
‖None of the growth-retarding factors in Table 3-1 in their pregnancies.

TABLE 15–14. — PREGNANCY OUTCOME AMONG BLACK CONTROL PRIMIPARAS ACCORDING TO THEIR AGES

MATERNAL AGE, YEARS	INFANTS		FULL-TERM INFANTS			
	Total No.	< 37 wk No.	Total No.	LPI* No.	SHFD† No.	Small OF‡ circ. No.
25–20	79	3	76	3	10	5
19–17	93	4	89	4	12	5
< 17	41	1	40	4	3	4
Total	213	8(3.8%)	205	11(5.4%)	25(12.2%)	14(6.8%)

*LPI, low ponderal index (< fifth percentile, Table 4-5).
†SHFD, short-for-dates (≤ fifth percentile, Tables 15-1 and 15-2).
‡Small OF, occipitofrontal circumference (≤ fifth percentile, Tables 15-3 and 15-4).

ence between the latter and controls is statistically significant, $p < 0.01$. Full-term infants with low ponderal indices occurred more than twice as frequently among mothers with LWG as among control mothers. The incidence of short-for-dates (SHFD) infants among 63 mothers with LWG who had other behavioral conditions was 22.1% and was statistically significantly higher than among 497 control mothers, $p < 0.01$.

Black mothers who were considered underweight for their heights at conception had a particularly poor outcome of their pregnancies (Table 15–13). Incidences of premature infants and of full-term infants with low ponderal indices and of full-term infants who were short-for-dates were significantly higher among underweight mothers than among mothers who had no known growth-retarding factors in their pregnancies, p being < 0.05 in each instance. Half the mothers who were underweight had other behavioral conditions; their pregnancy outcome was comparable to that of mothers whose only known growth-retarding factor was their being underweight at conception.

Pregnancy outcome for primiparous black control mothers was unusual as compared to pregnancy outcome for comparable white mothers. Black control primiparas had a surprisingly high incidence (12.2%) of full-term SHFD infants (Table 15–14); the incidence of SHFD infants was high among teenage black primiparas and also among those 20–25 years of age. The incidence of SHFD infants born to black primiparas (12.2%) was almost 3 times higher than the incidence of 4.2% among 306 black control multiparas.

Pregnancy outcome among black mothers who were 35 years or more of age was comparable to that observed among older white mothers. Congenital malformations were observed among 3 of the 27 single infants born to black mothers; 1 infant had Down's syndrome, another had a double thumb and the third had a tetralogy of Fallot. Fifteen of the 27 mothers had no known growth-retarding factors in their pregnancies and none of their infants had low ponderal indices or small occipitofrontal circumferences or were short-for-dates; 1 infant was born before 37 completed weeks of gestation. Among the 9 infants born to 9 mothers with behavioral conditions, 1 was prematurely born, 3 were short-for-dates and 3 had small occipitofrontal circumferences.

There were 17 black mothers who had no prenatal care. There were 5 premature infants and 2 short-for-dates full-term infants born to the group of 17 mothers. The high incidence of premature and short-for-dates infants was also observed among white mothers with little or no prenatal care in Chapter 12.

REFERENCES
1. Sargent, D. W.: Weight-height relationship of young men and women, Am. J. Clin. Nutr. 13:318, 1963.
2. Miller, H. C., and Hassanein, K.: Diagnosis of impaired fetal growth in newborn infants, Pediatrics 48:511, 1971.

16 / Twin Pregnancies

THE HIGH INCIDENCE of fetal undergrowth among twins provides an excellent opportunity for studying fetal growth retardation (FGR) in all of its important forms. Even a small number of twins will demonstrate the different types of FGR and the occurrence of retarded fetal growth in some large infants whose birth weights were not low for their gestational ages.

Data presented in this chapter concern 37 sets of white twins born consecutively at The University of Kansas Medical Center. Twins in 17 of the 37 sets were born prematurely (< 37 completed weeks of gestation); 32 of the 34 twins born prematurely had birth weights under 2500 gm. Many of the 34 premature twins probably were undergrown in utero. Their birth weights, including those premature twins whose mothers had no other known growth-retarding factors in their pregnancies, were lower than the birth weights of premature singleton infants of similar gestational ages born to control mothers (Fig. 4–12) and corresponded closely to the birth weights of premature singletons (Fig. 4–14) who were born to mothers with medical complications and behavioral conditions in their pregnancies.

The group of 20 sets of full-term twins provided striking evidence of fetal undergrowth; 11 of the 40 full-term twins had birth weights under 2500 gm. Three of the sets had uncertain gestational dates, leaving 17 sets for purposes of this study. Severe FGR (≤ fifth percentiles) was observed in crown-heel lengths, head circumferences, ponderal indices and birth weights in all but 2 of the 17 sets. Both twins in 10 sets had evidence of FGR and 1 twin in each of the 5 remaining sets had evidence of FGR. The percentiles of growth attained at birth by the twins in the 17 sets are shown in Table 16–1. Their attained growth at birth in height, head circumference, weight and ponderal index is compared to that of full-term control singletons born to mothers with no known growth-retarding factors in their

TABLE 16–1.–ATTAINED PERCENTILES OF GROWTH
AT BIRTH IN 17 SETS OF WHITE FULL-TERM TWINS

PERCENTILE OF ATTAINED GROWTH	INFANTS			
	Birth weight*	Crown-heel† length	Occipito‡ frontal circ.	Ponderal index§
	No.	No.	No.	No.
76–90	1	1	2	1
51–75	1	1	2	4
26–50	4	5	5	2
11–25	3	6	7	4
6–10	4	3	6	2
≤ 5	21	17	11	11
N.D.	-	1	1	1
Total	34	34	34	25‖

*Birth weights according to percentiles in Tables 4-11, 4-12, 4-13 and 4-14.
†Crown-heel lengths according to percentiles in Tables 4-2 and 4-3.
‡Occipitofrontal circumferences according to percentiles in Tables 4-7 and 4-8.
§Ponderal indices according to percentiles for multipara in Table 4-5.
‖Calculated for twins with body lengths ≥ 48.5 cm only.

pregnancies. Data on attained growth at birth of full-term control infants are shown in tables in Chapter 4. Five per cent of control singletons are expected to be at the fifth percentiles and 50% to be at the fiftieth percentiles. It can be seen in Table 16–1 that 21 (over 60%) of the 34 twins had birth weights at or below the fifth percentile in accordance with their sex and gestational ages and parity (primipara or multipara) of their mothers; 17 of the 34 twins had crown-heel lengths at or below the fifth percentile for their sex and gestational ages; 11 of 34 twins had occipitofrontal circumferences at or below the fifth percentile for their sex and gestational ages; 11 of 25 twins whose crown-heel lengths were 48.5 cm or more had ponderal indices at or below the fifth percentile. There were 9 in the group of 34 twins who had no evidence of severe fetal growth retardation (≤fifth percentile). Few of the 34 twins attained growth above the fiftieth percentiles in any of the four parameters.

The largest intrapair differences in full-term twins were observed in their birth weights. Intrapair differences in crown-heel lengths and head circumferences were much less than differences in birth weights. In the set of twins with the largest difference in birth weights, the heavier twin's weight exceeded the lighter twin's by 41.5%. The largest intrapair difference in crown-heel lengths was in a set in which the body length of the longer twin exceeded the length of the shorter twin by 7.5%. The largest intrapair difference in head circumferences was in a set in which the circumference of the head of the larger twin exceeded that of the smaller twin by 10%. The largest intrapair differences in ponderal indices in any set of twins was 25%.

Full-term twins whose birth weights were at or below the fifth percentiles for their gestational age, sex and maternal parity exhibited various combinations of severe growth retardation in body lengths, head circumferences and ponderal indices. Some of these combinations are illustrated by data in Table 16–2. The 5 sets of full-term twins in Table 16–2 were born to mothers who had no known growth-retarding factors in their pregnancies of the types listed in Table 3–1 except the factor of multiple birth. All 10 twins had moderate to severe retardation of growth in one or more parameters. There was only 1 of the 10 twins (number 2 in case 3) that did not have at least one parameter at or below the fifth percentile and the crown-heel length of that twin was at the

TABLE 16–2.—BIRTH DATA ON 5 SETS OF FULL-TERM TWINS BORN TO WHITE MOTHERS WITH NO OTHER KNOWN GROWTH-RETARDING FACTORS* IN THEIR PREGNANCIES

CASE NO.		FETAL AGE, WEEKS	SEX	BIRTH WEIGHT, GM	PONDERAL INDEX	CROWN-HEEL LENGTH, CM	HEAD CIRC., CM
1	MZ	39	F	2357†	2.20	47.5†	31.9†
			F	2626†	2.37	48.0†	32.0†
2	DZ	42	M	2996†	2.19†	51.5	34.7
			M	3278	2.19†	53.0	34.3
3	MZ	40	M	2486†	2.46	46.5†	34.4
			M	3152	2.52	50.0	36.0
4	?DZ	39	M	2914	2.23†	50.5	33.0†
			M	2586†	2.07†	50.0	32.8†
5	DZ	42	F	2895†	2.39	49.5†	34.6
			F	2856†	2.28	50.0†	33.6†

*Growth-retarding factors listed in Table 3-1.
† ≤ Fifth percentile for control singleton infants, Chapter 4.
MZ = monozygotic; DZ = dizygotic.

tenth percentile. Seven of the 10 twins had birth weights at or below the fifth percentile and all of the remaining 3 twins had birth weights that were below the twenty-fifth percentile for singletons; 2 of the 3 twins whose birth weights were above the fifth percentile had markedly reduced ponderal indices (< fifth percentile), indicating that birth weight is not an ideal parameter for evaluating fetal growth retardation.

There were no clues in the histories of the mothers of the twins as to the types of fetal growth retardation that were observed. Twins in Table 16–2 were labeled as monozygotic or dizygotic after gross and microscopic examinations of the chorions and amnions and after determination of their blood groups. Twins with a single chorion and two amnions and having identical blood groups were labeled as monozygotic.

There were 5 sets of twins born to mothers who reported smoking 10 or more cigarettes a day. Two of the 5 mothers had other behavioral conditions in their pregnancies. None of the 5 mothers had other growth-retarding factors listed in Table 3–1. The 10 twins in these 5 sets had even a greater incidence of severe fetal growth retardation than the twins born to mothers shown in Table 16–2. Nine of the 10 twins had birth weights at or below the fifth percentile; 7 of the 10 had crown-heel lengths at or below the fifth percentile.

Previous reports on the growth of twins suggest that their retarded growth in utero begins at the start of the third trimester of pregnancy.[1-4] Naeye and associates[4] observed that dichorionic twins did not show evidence of retarded growth until about the thirty-fourth week of pregnancy. These reports were based on comparisons of the birth weights of twins with the birth weights of singletons of comparable gestational ages. Our study of singleton premature infants reported in Chapter 4 suggests that most of them have been born to mothers who had growth-retarding factors in their pregnancies, especially those born before the thirty-fourth week. It may be incorrect to compare premature twins with premature singletons on the assumption that the latter have been normally grown in utero, unless it can be shown that the singleton premature infants were born to mothers free from all known growth-retarding factors. It is possible that the onset of retarded somatic growth in twins occurs much earlier in pregnancy than previously believed.

Studies of postnatal growth of twins indicate that the smaller twins in sets that differed in birth weights by 36% on the average remained smaller in height, weight and head circumference during the first 10–13 years after birth[5] and that twins in general weighed less and were shorter than singletons at 2 years of age.[6] There is need for studies of the postnatal growth of twins whose prenatal growth in body length, weight and head size has been diagnosed at or before birth by appropriate techniques. Twins provide an especially high incidence of the various types of fetal undergrowth and some sets of twins also provide the opportunity to compare a particular type of fetal undergrowth in one twin with a more normal growth in the other twin.

REFERENCES
1. McKeown, T., and Record, R. G.: Observations on foetal growth in multiple pregnancy in man, J. Endocrinol. 8:386, 1952.
2. Guttmacher, A. F., and Schuyler, K. G.: The fetus of multiple gestations, Obstet. Gynecol. 12:528, 1958.
3. Naeye, R. L.: The fetal and neonatal development of twins, Pediatrics 33:546, 1964.
4. Naeye, R. L., Benirschke, K., Hagstrom, W. C., and Marcus, C. C.: Intrauterine growth of twins as estimated from liveborn birth-weight data, Pediatrics 37:409, 1966.
5. Babson, S. G., and Phillips, D. S.: Growth and development of twins dissimilar in size at birth, N. Engl. J. Med. 289:937, 1973.
6. Chamberlain, R., and Davey, A.: Physical growth in twins, postmature and small-for-dates children, Arch. Dis. Child. 50:437, 1975.

17 / Prenatal and Postnatal Growth: Is There a Continuum?

RECENT REPORTS suggest that there is a continuum of prenatal and postnatal growth, but the degree and extent to which prenatal growth affects postnatal growth continues to be debated. Garn and associates[1] state that the most important single determinant of individual growth during the first 7 postnatal years for normal term infants is their body size (weight, length, head circumference) at birth. Smith's group[2] reported on 90 normal full-term infants, two-thirds of whom shifted their growth curves for height either upward or downward by one or more percentile lines by 2 years of age. Percentile lines were established by Smith's group at third, tenth, twenty-fifth, fiftieth, seventy-fifth, ninetieth and ninety-seventh percentiles. Two-thirds of the 90 infants had an upward shift of their heights across one or more percentile lines in the first 3 postnatal months. This high incidence of upward shifts in the first 3 postnatal months may have partly depended on an artifact relating to the infants' gestational ages at birth. The postnatal growth chart developed by Smith's group assumes that all 90 infants had the same gestational age. Gestational age has a marked effect on the percentile of height an infant is placed on at birth. For example, in Table 4–2, full-term male infants 50.5 cm long at 37 weeks of gestation are on the seventy-fifth percentile for height, on the twenty-fifth percentile if they are at 39 weeks and at the fifth percentile if their gestational age is 42 weeks. We have found at The University of Kansas Medical Center that there is much less shifting across percentile lines in infants' heights during the first few postnatal months if their heights are plotted at birth according to their gestational ages. There is some upward and downward shifting across percentile lines for height even after allowance has been made for gestational age at birth. However, we have been impressed that full-term infants whose crown-heel lengths were short at birth for their gestational ages had good mean postnatal velocity growth in height but their mean heights at 1 and 2 years of age remained short.[3] Some short infants had a moderate upward shift and others had a downward shift or no shift in height percentiles during the first 2 years. Fitzhardinge and Steven[4] examined the growth in height of a group of full-term infants whose birth weights were more than 2 standard deviations below the mean for that particular nursery. The body lengths of these infants at birth generally, but not always, were at or below 48 cm and most of the infants probably would fit our diagnosis of short-for-dates; a few of their infants with longer body lengths at birth probably would fit our diagnosis of a malnourished infant with a low ponderal index. The group as a whole was heterogeneous for height at birth. Their postnatal growth was plotted on charts designed by Stuart and Reed[5] that make no allowance for gestational age. The mean attained growth in heights for boys and girls studied by Fitzhardinge and Steven proceeded along the lower percentiles for height. The mean attained height for girls at 5 years of age was at the third percentile and at 8 years of age was below the third percentile. Boys fared a little better. Their mean attained growth in height at 4 years was at the third percentile and at 8 years was at about the fifteenth to twentieth percentiles.

One of the problems in most previous reports of follow-up studies on newborn infants is the inability of the reader to distinguish between the different types of fetal growth retardation present at birth, because investigators relied so heavily on a low birth weight for gestational age to diagnose fetal undergrowth. We judge that most full-term infants diagnosed as undergrown in utero on the basis of a low birth weight for gestational age probably are short-for-dates. Cruise[6] observed that full-term infants with birth weights under 2500 gm were shorter at 1, 2 and 3 years of age than full-term infants over 2500 gm at birth. Velocity growth in heights during the first 3 years appeared to be comparable in the two groups of full-term infants.

We have observed that some tall infants whose body lengths at birth in The University of Kansas Medical Center were at or above the ninetieth percentile for their gestational ages had a downward shift in percentiles for height in the first 2 postnatal years whereas others maintained growth in height on the high percentiles on which they were born.

One of the questions that has not been resolved about growth in height during the early postnatal years is why some infants shift upward, others shift downward and some maintain their heights. Smith's group postulates that body length at birth relates mainly to maternal size (height) and at 2 years of age length relates best to mean parental height, reflecting the genetic growth factors of both parents. It would be interesting to learn what the differences in incidence of infants who had shifts in height percentiles in their study would have been had they plotted body lengths at birth according to percentiles for gestational ages and not on the assumption that all 90 infants were of the same gestational age. Upward and downward shifts in height in the early postnatal years probably is multifactorial. One of the factors almost certainly is the infant's nutritional status. Infants who are undernourished over sufficiently long periods exhibit some growth retardation in their heights. Forbes[7] found that children who became obese exhibited a distinct tendency for growth in height to accelerate coincident with or after the onset of excessive weight gain. We have observed the same phenomenon in infants. In our studies of prenatal and postnatal growth at The University of Kansas Medical Center, infants who maintained their growth in height on the same or higher percentiles than the one on which they were born also maintained their growth in weight on the same or higher percentiles.[8] Downward shifts in percentiles for height frequently were preceded by drop-offs in percentiles for weight; explanations for the drop-offs in weight were not clearly established.

The postnatal growth of malnourished full-term infants at The University of Kansas Medical Center has been different from that of the short-for-dates infants.[3] The malnourished infants had slightly reduced crown-heel lengths at birth that were within normal limits for their gestational ages; they had low ponderal indices and low weight-height ratios.[9] Naeye[10] observed that the livers, spleens, thymus and adrenal glands of malnourished newborn infants weighed less than those of well-nourished infants. Naeye and his associates[11, 12] agree with Gruenwald and others that this type of undergrowth arises late in gestation. In our experience, newborn infants who fit these criteria developed large appetites, accelerated their weight gains beginning shortly after birth and usually caught up in weight to full-term infants who had normal fetal growth by the age of 3–6 months. In the few malnourished infants who did not accelerate their weight gains after birth, we found some cause for their failure to accelerate. Either there had been physical illness or some psychosocial factor, such as inability of the mother to cope because of her emotional or mental status or because of child abuse or some mechanical factor, such as an inappropriate nipple in an infant fed artificially. Malnourished newborn infants sometimes had accelerated gains in height coincident with their accelerated weight gains. Once they had caught up to infants normally grown in utero, they continued to grow along the new percentiles during the first 2 postnatal years. Follow-up studies on these infants beyond the second year are in progress.

Fetuses accumulate fat during the third trimester of pregnancy and some of them are born obese. The relationship between obesity acquired during the third trimester and subsequent obesity in infancy and early childhood is not clear. Most studies of obese infants and young children have been based on birth data collected retrospectively and sometimes limited to a single parameter—birth weight—or based on velocity of weight gain during infancy. There is need for studies in which obesity in newborn infants is diagnosed prospectively by proper criteria, including physical appearance, weight-height ratios or indices or ponderal indices and measurements of skin-fold thickness and in which follow-up examinations are made with care in order to evaluate the many factors associated with the development of obesity. Fisch and his associates[13] made use of data collected at the Minnesota site as part of the Collaborative Perinatal Project of the National Institutes of Health. Data collected at birth and 4 and 7 years of age revealed that neonates with a high weight to height index (> ninety-fifth percentile) tended to retain heavy physiques for at least the first 7 years after birth. Those infants who became very obese by 4 years of age were likely to retain heavy physiques up to 7 years of age. Data on growth during the interim periods were not available. Studies by Eid[14] suggested that excessive weight gains by infants in the first 6 postnatal months were associated with significant increases in the incidence of obese children from 6 to 8 years of age when compared to infants who had lesser weight gains in the first 6 months. Brook and associates[15] observed an increased size and number of fat cells in infants who gained excessive weight and had weights above the ninety-fifth percentile at 1 year of age. On the other hand, Mellbin and Vuille[16] found questionable evidence in girls and possibly a little evidence in boys that an increased velocity of weight gain in infancy was significantly associated with an increased incidence of children who were overweight at 7 years of age.

We favor an increased velocity of weight gain in infants who are born malnourished and have low ponderal indices at birth, so that they can recover quickly from their malnourished state and catch up in weight to infants who have had normal fetal growth. The matter of preventing obesity in infancy and childhood solely by dietary measures instituted early in infancy remains controversial in view of the conflicting results cited above concerning the effects of accelerated weight gains on the subsequent development of obesity and in view of the many other factors that need to be taken into account in the development of obesity, including physical activity, familial and genetic background and psychosocial factors. Fomon and Ziegler[17] provide additional factors with which to be concerned in the matter of preventing obesity in children. They warn that there is no satisfactory medical definition of obesity in children and that moderate degrees of obesity may allow some individuals to function optimally whereas the same degree of obesity in another person may be a health hazard.

It appears that the extent and degree to which postnatal growth is a continuum of different patterns of prenatal growth have not been studied as thoroughly as they might be. There is need for more prospective studies that would provide clinicians with better insight into an interesting and important area of somatic growth.

REFERENCES

1. Garn, S. M., Shaw, H. A., and McCabe, K. D.: Birth size and growth appraisal, J. Pediatr. 90:1049, 1977.
2. Smith, D. W., Truog, W., Rogers, J. E., Greitzer, L. J., Skinner, A. L., McCann, J. J., and Henry, M. A. S.: Shifting linear growth during infancy: Illustration of genetic factors in growth from fetal life through infancy, J. Pediatr. 89:225, 1976.

3. Holmes, G. E., Miller, H. C., Hassanein, K., Lansky, S., and Goggin, J. E.: Postnatal somatic growth in infants with atypical fetal growth patterns, Am. J. Dis. Child. 131:1078, 1977.
4. Fitzhardinge, P. M., and Steven, E. M.: The small-for-date infant. 1. Later growth patterns, Pediatrics 49:671, 1972.
5. Stuart, H. C., and Reed, R. B.: Longitudinal studies of child health and development, Pediatrics (supp.) 24:875, 1959.
6. Cruise, M. O.: A longitudinal study of the growth of low birth weight infants, Pediatrics 51:620, 1973.
7. Forbes, G. B.: Nutrition and growth, J. Pediatr. 91:40, 1977.
8. Holmes, G. E., and Miller, H. C.: Unpublished studies.
9. Miller, H. C., and Hassanein, K.: Diagnosis of impaired fetal growth in newborn infants, Pediatrics 48:511, 1971.
10. Naeye, R. L.: Malnutrition, probable cause of fetal growth retardation, Arch. Pathol. 79:284, 1965.
11. Naeye, R. L., Blanc, W., and Paul, C.: Effects of maternal nutrition on the human fetus, Pediatrics 52:494, 1973.
12. Gruenwald, P.: Chronic fetal distress and placental insufficiency, Biol. Neonate 5:215, 1963.
13. Fisch, R. O., Bilek, M. K., and Ulstron, R.: Obesity and leanness at birth and their relationship to body habitus in later childhood, Pediatrics 56:521, 1975.
14. Eid, E. E.: Follow-up study of physical growth of children who had excessive weight gain in the first 6 months of life, Br. Med. J. 2:74, 1970.
15. Brook, C. G. D., Lloyd, J. K., and Wolff, O. H.: Relation between age of onset of obesity and size and number of adipose cells, Br. Med. J. 2:25, 1972.
16. Mellbin, T., and Vuille, J. C.: Physical development at 7 years of age in relation to velocity of weight gain in infancy with special reference to incidence of overweight, Br. J. Prev. Soc. Med. 27:225, 1973.
17. Fomon, S. J., and Ziegler, E. E.: Prevention of Obesity. Nutritional Disorders of Children. U. S. Department of Health, Education, and Welfare. DHEW Publication No. (HSA) 76-5612. Government Printing Office, Washington, D. C., 1976.

18 / Ultrasonic Measurements

ULTRASONIC MEASUREMENTS of fetal parts have provided much useful information about fetal maturity, fetal growth and, in some instances, fetal size. There seems to be general agreement that ultrasonic measurements of the fetal biparietal diameter can be highly reliable when made by one who is experienced and expert in using the technique and that good estimates of gestational age can be made from these measurements if they are done at the proper time.[1-3] Campbell[1] reported that the optimal period for estimating gestational age from biparietal measurements was between the 20th and 30th weeks of pregnancy. Sabbagha et al.[3] agreed on the period from 20 to 28 weeks, because they found that linear regression analysis was applicable only during the period from 20 to 28 weeks.[3] During this period, fetal age for a given biparietal diameter varied by a maximum of ± 11 days from the mean in 95% of the population.

Investigators encountered difficulties when they attempted to estimate the body weights of newborn infants from single ultrasonic measurements of fetal biparietal diameters. Sabbagha,[4] in comparing results obtained by several different investigators, observed that fetal weight ranged from a low of ± 638 gm to a high of ± 980 gm at a given biparietal diameter in 95% of the populations studied. These wide ranges of body weight offered no additional advantages over older clinical methods, involving external measurements of fundal height of the uterus or palpation of the fetus through the abdominal wall. Such wide ranges of body weight for a given biparietal diameter could have been predicted, because much of the weight of a term fetus is dependent on soft tissue mass and the latter varies markedly depending on whether the fetus is well nourished and fat or poorly nourished and lean. As shown in Chapter 1, body weights of term infants may not correlate well with body sizes at birth. Measurements of external body dimensions provide a better method for evaluating body size. They are less affected by factors that retard fetal growth than are birth weights. Measurements of head circumference are even less affected than measurements of crown-heel length by the normal as well as unfavorable fetal growth factors. Biparietal diameters correlate with occipitofrontal circumferences and should provide helpful information in evaluations of cephalopelvic disproportions. Biparietal diameters and occipitofrontal circumferences correlate with crown-heel lengths.[5] Scammon and Calkins reported that for each increment in crown-heel length of 10 mm, occipitofrontal circumferences increased by 6 mm during the fetal period.

It now has become apparent that serial measurements of fetal body parts offer a better opportunity than single measurements for evaluating the dynamics of fetal growth. One of the important goals of present-day clinicians is to diagnose fetal growth retardation and fetal overgrowth during pregnancy. More rapid progress toward this goal will be achieved when clinicians appreciate that there are at least two main types of fetal growth retardation and that body weight in relation to gestational age cannot differentiate between the two types, as described in Chapter 1. Fetuses with either of the two types of fetal growth retardation may have the same birth weight. The long, lean fetus usually will have a head size that is proportionate to the normal crown-heel length for fetal age and the symmetrically retarded fetus will have a small head size that is commensurate with the short crown-heel length for fetal age. Campbell,[6] using serial ultrasonic measurements of fetal biparietal diameters, has observed fetal growth patterns that appear to distinguish between the two types of fetal growth retardation (Figs. 18–1 and 18–2). Figure 18–1 depicts the serial biparietal diameters of a long, lean infant who at birth had a low weight-height ratio or a low ponderal index. Figure 18–2 depicts the symmetrically small infant who fits our criteria for a short-for-dates (SHFD) infant. Attempts in the United States to use serial measurements of biparietal diameters routinely in the diagnosis of fetal growth retardation have not met with much success.[7] Campbell and Thoms[8] more recently have combined serial ultrasound measurements of biparietal diameters with single ultrasound measurements of the fetal head to abdomen circumference ratio in their assessment of growth

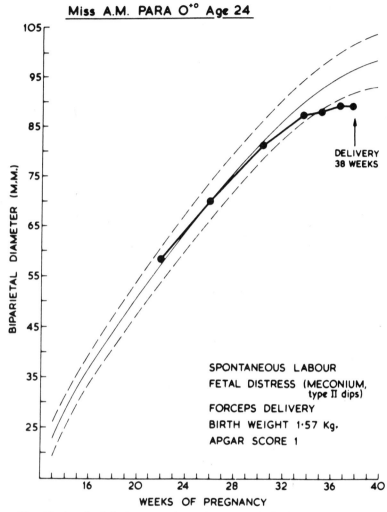

Fig. 18–1.—Serial ultrasound measurements of biparietal diameters in a fetus with "late flattening" pattern of growth retardation. Reproduced, with permission, from Stuart Campbell: Fetal growth, Clin. Obstet. Gynaecol. 1:41, 1974, by W. B. Saunders Company, Ltd.

retardation. They believe that the combination of measurements provides a better evaluation of fetal growth retardation than serial measurements of biparietal diameters alone. Unfortunately, they made the diagnosis of growth retardation at birth on the basis of a low birth weight for gestational age and did not provide

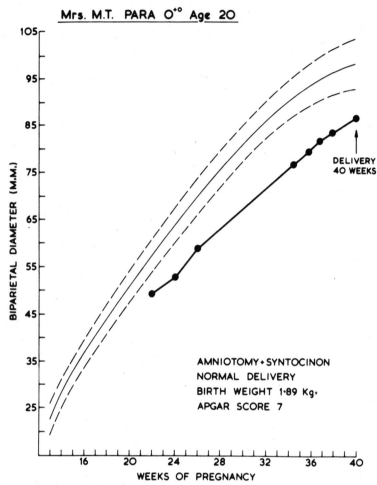

Fig. 18–2.—Serial ultrasound measurements of biparietal diameters in a fetus with a "low-profile" pattern of growth retardation. Reproduced, with permission, from Stuart Campbell: Fetal growth, Clin. Obstet. Gynaecol. 1:41, 1974, by W. B. Saunders Company, Ltd.

routine data on birth weights, lengths or head circumferences of the infants they diagnosed prenatally as growth retarded; consequently, it is not clear as to whether or not they were diagnosing one or two different types of fetal growth retardation. As we have mentioned before in this text, the symmetrically undergrown fetus whom we diagnose as short-for-dates may either appear lean and lacking in subcutaneous fat or appear well nourished and well supplied with subcutaneous fat. The short-for-dates infant is distinguished from infants with the other type of growth retardation, because the latter have normal crown-heel lengths for their gestational ages and invariably are lean. We believe that the latter infants have a much milder form of growth retardation that comes on much later in pregnancy than is the case with the short-for-dates infants.

Serial ultrasonic measurements of fetal biparietal diameters can be used to determine the rate at which the biparietal diameter is growing. Details of the method for diagnosing the growth rate of the fetal biparietal diameter are provided in an article by Campbell and Dewhurst.[9] When the growth rate of fetal biparietal diameters fell below the fifth percentile, they observed that 82% of babies were below the tenth percentile of weight for gestational age and 68% were below the fifth percentile of weight. This method will not diagnose all undergrown fetuses, because some fetuses who are symmetrically small for their gestational ages almost certainly will have normal growth rates of their biparietal diameters. Also, the fetus with a normal crown-heel length for gestational age and a reduced soft tissue mass usually has a normal growth rate in head size and in biparietal diameter.

Better estimates of fetal weight have been made by using ultrasonic measurements of the circumference of the fetal abdomen[10] and of the circumference of the fetal trunk.[11] Campbell and Wilkin[10] reported that a single measurement of the circumference of the abdomen at 32 weeks would detect 85% of infants whose birth weights were below the fifth percentile for their gestational ages and that this rate would fall to 68% at 38 weeks. Measurements of the circumference of the fetal trunk predicted birth weights obtained not later than 48 hours after the measurements with a mean prediction error of only 75 gm. Higginbottom's group[11] found that serial measurement of the circumference of the trunk was useful in monitoring fetal growth retardation. Campbell recommended that the diagnosis of fetal undergrowth be based on an early determination of fetal maturity using ultrasonic measurements of embryonic crown-rump length between 6 and 12 weeks, as suggested by Robinson,[12] and of biparietal diameters between 13 and 20 weeks, as suggested

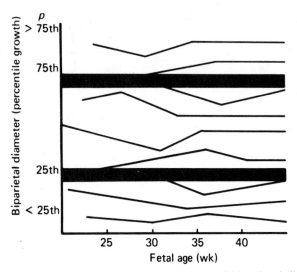

Fig. 18–3.—Serial ultrasound measurements of biparietal diameters of human fetuses, illustrating their tendency to maintain their cephalic rank during the last half of pregnancy. (From Sabbagha, R. E., Barton, B. A., Barton, F. B., et al.: Sonar biparietal diameter: II. Predictive of three fetal growth patterns leading to a closer assessment of gestational age and neonatal weight, Am. J. Obstet. Gynecol. 126:485–490, 1976. Reproduced with permission of the C. V. Mosby Company.)

by Campbell[13] in combination with a late measurement between 32 and 36 weeks of the circumference of the fetal abdomen.

We believe that it is important to differentiate between the two main types of fetal undergrowth. Their pathogeneses probably are different; their prenatal and postnatal courses are different.[14] The differential diagnosis between these two types of retarded growth is constantly made in older infants by using measurements of height and weight in relation to age. Sabbagha's studies suggest that the size of the fetus and of the newborn infant may be determined early in pregnancy.[4] Biparietal diameters do correlate directly with crown-heel length. He has shown (Fig. 18–3) that biparietal diameters measured by ultrasound at about 20 weeks tend to maintain their relative cephalic rank throughout pregnancy. Fetuses with small biparietal diameters at 20 weeks usually have small biparietal diameters at 40 weeks. It would be of interest to know if crown-rump measurements made between 6 and 12 weeks have predictive value for crown-heel length at 40 weeks and for biparietal diameters. It seems reasonable to believe that ultrasonic techniques should be able to measure intrauterine growth in body dimensions and, it is hoped, distinguish the symmetrically small fetus from the other type of fetal undergrowth that is mainly related to retarded growth of soft tissues or wasting of soft tissues.

REFERENCES

1. Campbell, S.: The prediction of fetal maturity by ultrasonic measurement of the biparietal diameter, J. Obstet. Gynaecol. Br. Commonw. 75:568, 1969.
2. Willocks, J., and Dunswore, I. R.: Reassessment of gestational age and prediction of dysmaturity by ultrasonic fetal cephalometry, J. Obstet. Gynaecol. Br. Commonw. 78:804, 1971.
3. Sabbagha, R. E., Turner, H. J., Rockette, H., et al.: Sonar BPD and fetal age definition of the relationship, Obstet. Gynecol. 43:7, 1974.
4. Sabbagha, R. E.: Biparietal diameter: An appraisal, Clin. Obstet. Gynaecol. 20:297, 1977.
5. Scammon, R. E., and Calkins, L. A.: Growth in the Fetal Period (Minneapolis: The University of Minnesota Press, 1929).
6. Campbell, S.: Fetal growth, Clin. Obstet. Gynaecol. 1:41, 1974.
7. Cooks, L. N.: Intrauterine and extrauterine recognition and management of deviant fetal growth, Pediatr. Clin. North Am. 24:431, 1977.
8. Campbell, S., and Thoms, A.: Ultrasound measurement of the fetal head to abdomen circumference ratio in the assessment of growth retardation, Br. J. Obstet. Gynaecol. 84:165, 1977.
9. Campbell, S., and Dewhurst, C. J.: Diagnosis of the small-for-dates fetus by serial ultrasonic cephalometry, Lancet 2:1202, 1971.
10. Campbell, S., and Wilkin, D.: Ultrasonic measurement of fetal abdomen circumference in the estimation of fetal weight, Br. J. Obstet. Gynaecol. 82:689, 1975.
11. Higginbottom, J., Slater, J., Porter, G., and Whitfield, C. R.: Br. J. Obstet. Gynaecol. 82:698, 1975.
12. Robinson, H.: Sonar measurement of fetal crown-rump length as means of assessing maturity in first trimester of pregnancy, Br. Med. J. 4:28, 1973.
13. Campbell, S.: Clinics in Perinatology, Vol. 1, No. 2, The Pregnancy at Risk, Milunsky, A. (ed.) (Philadelphia: W. B. Saunders Company, 1974).
14. Holmes, G. E., Miller, H. C., Hassanein, K., Lansky, S. B., and Goggin, J. E.: Postnatal somatic growth in infants with atypical fetal growth patterns, Am. J. Dis. Child. 131:1078, 1977.

19 / Other Prenatal Tests of Fetal Growth Retardation

INVESTIGATORS have shown great interest in developing laboratory tests that would detect atypical patterns of fetal growth in humans prior to birth. Their interest was not misplaced, in view of the strong correlation between fetal growth impairment and birth asphyxia, meconium aspiration, perinatal death, hypoglycemia, hypocalcemia, polycythemia and other perinatal conditions and their long-term consequences for survivors. Early prenatal diagnosis of fetal growth retardation and fetal overgrowth would be helpful in anticipating and, it is hoped, in avoiding these adversities. The incidence of fetal growth retardation in humans has not been established. The incidence obviously depends on circumstances connected with pregnancies, as we have illustrated in preceding chapters, and also on the criteria used in its diagnosis. Recent estimates of incidence by the National Institute of Child Health and Human Development based only on birth weights under 2500 gm suggest that 2–3% of all pregnancies terminate with births of growth-retarded infants.[1] This probably is an underestimate.

The evaluation of fetal growth rests on the establishment of normal values and a correct diagnosis of fetal age. Establishing gestational age precisely on large numbers of infants is not without its errors. Investigators have attempted to provide what they considered were measurements of normal values for body weight, limb lengths, crown-rump lengths, biparietal diameters, head circumference and weights of various organs.[2-11] Unfortunately, few authors separated fetuses according to race or sex, and all calculations of gestational age were based on maternal recall of the last menstrual period. The number of fetuses at each week of gestation were also limited, making it impossible to determine with confidence percentile ranges in the first two trimesters of pregnancy.

The time of appearance of primary and and secondary centers of ossification in fetuses has been used to determine gestational ages, but the usefulness of radiographs obtained prenatally is seriously limited by difficulties in recording centers when present, because of poor fetal position or interference from maternal and fetal tissues.[12-14] It is interesting that Cruikshank and associates[12] observed in whole-body radiographs of infants at birth that their centers of ossification correlated best with body lengths. There is wide variation in the time of appearance of the distal femoral and proximal tibial epiphyses that depends not only on sex and race but also on fetal undernutrition and the state of endocrine control over their appearance. Scott and Usher[15] found that these two centers were lacking in 37% of "malnourished" infants (25% underweight for gestational age) and significantly smaller in those deemed "malnourished" for age. If these two centers can be correctly diagnosed as present in a fetus, the likelihood is great that the fetus is at term.

Infants with intrauterine growth retardation have been observed to have a diminished fetal zone in their adrenal glands at birth. Levels of serum cortisol, 16-α-hydroxyepiandrosterone and dehydroepisandrosterone sulfate are significantly lower in these infants.[16-19] These steroids are the major contributors to estrogens appearing in maternal sera and urine. Diminished amounts of the fetal precursors of maternal estrogens may partially explain the reduced levels of plasma and urinary levels of estriol observed in mothers of growth-retarded newborn infants. Several investigators have suggested that the amount of estriol in maternal urine may be useful in establishing the adequacy of fetal growth and well-being.[20-23] Others have found that only 60–84% of infants with low birth weights for their gestational ages could be predicted by low amounts of estriols in maternal urine collected over a period of 24 hours.[24-26] They also reported a false positive rate of 20%. Some investigators have attempted to predict fetal growth retardation using serum levels of estriols and estradiol or plasma levels of estrogen.[27] To date, correlations among these blood levels have been less impressive than determining the amount of estriol in a 24-hour collection of urine.[28, 29] Campbell and Kurjak[30] reported a poor correlation between assays of urinary estrogen and the assessment of fetal growth retardation by serial ultrasonic cephalometry. If further studies of maternal estrogen levels in relation to fetal growth are to be undertaken, it would seem essential that the types of fetal growth retardation be taken into account. This has not been done in previous studies of the problem.

Human placental lactogen (hPL) has also been used in the biochemical assessment of fetal growth deficiency. Spellacy and associates[31] reported decreased serum levels of hPL in mothers delivered of growth-retarded newborn infants in nearly all instances. It is interesting that maternal levels of hPL are more closely correlated with placental weight than with fetal weight. Hensleigh and his group[32] combined determinations of oxytocinase and hPL. They reported that they could identify nearly 75% of fetuses who were developing intrauterine growth retardation from low sera levels of oxytocinase and hPL. The frequency of false positive and false negative results in their study diminishes the usefulness of their test. Furthermore, they did not distinguish between the different types of fetal growth retardation, and by using a low birth weight for fetal age to diagnose retarded fetal growth, they missed growth-retarded fetuses whose birth weights exceeded their arbitrarily selected cutoff birth weights.

Other biochemical markers of fetal growth retardation that have been tested prior to birth are remarkably few, and, in most instances, are indirect determinants. Rosado and associates were unable to find placental metabolic markers, including assays of pyruvic kinase, adenylate kinase and protein/DNA ratios, that could distinguish between several different groups of infants, some of whom were full-term and growth retarded in utero as judged by their weights, lengths and head circumferences and some of whom were premature infants with birth weights below 2.5 kg and above the tenth percentile for their gestational ages and judged to have appropriate birth weights for their gestational ages.[33, 34] Comprehensive studies of the metabolic activities of maternal leukocytes during the latter part of term pregnancies have been reported by Metcoff and associates.[35-37] Their results suggest that mothers delivering infants with fetal malnutrition have significantly lower values for pyruvic kinase and adenylate kinase in their leukocytes in peripheral blood at the time of delivery. Crosby *et al.*,[38] in 182 women, found significant differences at midgestation in total carotene, plasma zinc, alpha-1-globulin and ten amino acids (aspartic acid, threonine, serine, leucine, tyrosine, phenylalanine, lysine, histidine, arginine, ornithine) in maternal serum and leukocytes in women whose pregnancy resulted in an infant with a low "adjusted birth weight." However, actual variations in fetal growth abnormalities were not identified in this study. These workers conclude, "It is likely that analyses of the metabolic pattern of the maternal leukocyte during pregnancy may predict fetal malnutrition."[38] The application of their research to general routine clinical use has yet to be made. It is hoped that their observations will aid in differentiating between fetuses who are symmetrically reduced in body dimensions and fetuses of normal body size who have unusually low ratios of body weight to body length.

Fetal growth and maturity are not necessarily parallel, especially in complicated pregnancies. Evaluation of fetal size and growth may be misleading in estimating functional maturity of the lungs in terms of surfactant production. Changes in the concentrations of phospholipids in amniotic fluid (derived from fetal lung effluent) increase and decrease in a highly predictable fashion in normal pregnancies as gestation proceeds. Normally, surface-active phosphatidylcholine first appears in the amniotic fluid at about 24–26 weeks. Sphingomyelin, although found slightly earlier than phosphatidylcholine, continues to rise beyond 35 weeks' gestation.[39] Associated with these biochemical changes, anatomic maturation of the fetal lung proceeds from cylindrical tubular airways to the more spherical alveoli characteristic of mature lungs. The L/S ratio and, more recently, the Lung Profile are clinical evaluations used to document functional maturity of the lung, especially in pregnancies in which the fetus may have been exposed to numerous growth-altering stimuli, including diabetes mellitus, a variety of placental dysfunction syndromes and maternal conditions, including hypertension, endocrine imbalances and renal disease. Determination of functional maturity by appropriate techniques often is necessary in situations in which alterations in fetal growth and maturation of the fetal lung do not always coincide.

REFERENCES

1. Little Babies, Born Too Soon, Born Too Small. National Institutes of Child Health and Human Development. DHEW Publication No. (NIH) 77-1079.
2. Potter, E. L., and Craig, J. M.: Rate of Antenatal Growth, in *Pathol-*

ogy of the Fetus and the Infant (3d ed.; Chicago: Year Book Medical Publishers, Inc., 1975), p. 15.

3. Streeter, G. L.: Weight, sitting height, head size, foot length and menstrual age of the human embryo, Embryology 11:143, 1920.
4. Scammon, R. E., and Calkins, L. A.: *Growth in the Fetal Period* (Minneapolis: University of Minnesota Press, 1929).
5. Arey, L. B.: Correlation of fetal age and size, Am. J. Obstet. Gynecol. 54:872, 1947.
6. Scott, R. B., Jenkins, M. E., and Crawford, R. P.: Growth and development of Negro infants, Pediatrics 6:425, 1950.
7. Baumgartner, L.: Weight in relation to fetal and newborn mortality: Influence of sex and color, Pediatrics 6:329, 1950.
8. Schultz, D. M., Giordano, D. A., and Schultz, D. H.: Weights of organs of fetuses and infants, Arch. Pathol. 74:244, 1962.
9. Gruenwald, P.: Growth of the human fetus, Am. J. Obstet. Gynecol. 94:1112, 1966.
10. Yerushalmy, J.: Relation of birth weight, gestational age and the rate of intrauterine growth to perinatal mortality, Clin. Obstet. Gynaecol. 13:107, 1970.
11. Milner, R. D. G., and Richards, B.: An analysis of birth weight by gestational age of infants born in England and Wales, 1967–1971, J. Obstet. Gynaecol. Br. Commonw. 81:956, 1974.
12. Cruikshank, J. N., Miller, M. J., and Browne, F. J.: The estimation of foetal age, the weight and length of normal foetuses, and weights of foetal organs, Med. Res. Counc. Rep. Ser. No. 86, His Majesty's Stationery Office, London, 1924.
13. Christie, A.: Prevalence and distribution of ossification centers in newborn infant, Am. J. Dis. Child. 77:355, 1949.
14. Berridge, F. R., and Eton, B.: Accuracy of radiological estimation of foetal maturity, J. Obstet. Gynaecol. Br. Emp. 65:625, 1958.
15. Scott, K. E., and Usher, R.: Epiphyseal development in fetal malnutrition syndrome, N. Engl. J. Med. 270:822, 1964.
16. Kenny, F. M., and Preeyasombat, C.: Cortisol production rate. VI. Hypoglycemia in the neonatal and postnatal period and in association with dwarfism, J. Pediatr. 70:65, 1967.
17. Reynolds, J. W., and Murkin, B. L.: Urinary steroid levels in newborn infants with intrauterine growth retardation, J. Clin. Endocrinol. Metab. 36:576, 1973.
18. Cleary, R. E., Depp, R., and Pion, R.: Relation of C_{19} steroid sulfates in cord plasma to maternal urinary estriol, Am. J. Obstet. Gynecol. 106:534, 1970.
19. Turnipseed, M. R., Bentley, K., and Reynolds, J. W.: Serum dehydroepiandrosterone sulfate in premature infants and infants with intrauterine growth retardation, J. Clin. Endocrinol. Metab. 43:1219, 1976.
20. Easterling, W. E., and Talbert, L. M.: Estriol excretion in normal and complicated pregnancies, Am. J. Obstet. Gynecol. 107:417, 1970.

21. Martin, J. D., Hahnel, R., Kean, B. P., and Troy, V. G.: Urinary oestrogen excretion in women with intrauterine fetal growth retardation, Aust. N. Z. J. Obstet. Gynaecol. 12:102, 1972.
22. Klopper, A.: The assessment of fetoplacental function by estriol assay, Obstet. Gynecol. Surv. 23:813, 1968.
23. Bergsjo, D., Bakke, T., Salamonsen, L. A., Stoa, K. L., and Thorson, T.: Urinary oestriol in pregnancy, daily fluctuation and correlation with fetal growth, J. Obstet. Gynaecol. Br. Commonw. 80:305, 1973.
24. Galbraith, R. S., Low, J. A., and Boston, R. W.: Maternal urinary estriol excretion pattern in patients with chronic fetal insufficiency, Am. J. Obstet. Gynecol. 106:352, 1970.
25. Michne, E. A.: Urinary oestriol excretion in pregnancies complicated by suspected retarded intrauterine growth, toxaemia or essential hypertension, J. Obstet. Gynaecol. Br. Commonw. 74:986, 1967.
26. Elliott, P. M.: Urinary oestriol excretion in retarded intrauterine fetal growth, Aust. N. Z. J. Obstet. Gynaecol. 10:18, 1970.
27. Aickin, D. R., Smith, M. A., and Brown, J. B.: Comparison between plasma and urinary oestrogen measurements in predicting fetal risk, Aust. N. Z. J. Obstet. Gynaecol. 14:59, 1974.
28. Arias, F.: The diagnosis and management of intrauterine growth retardation, Obstet. Gynecol. 49:293, 1977.
29. Jones, M. D., and Battaglia, F. C.: Intrauterine growth retardation, Am. J. Obstet. Gynecol. 127:540, 1977.
30. Campbell, S., and Kurjak, A.: Comparison between urinary oestrogen assay and serial ultrasonic cephalometry in assessment of fetal growth retardation, Br. Med. J. 4:336, 1972.
31. Spellacy, W. N., Usategui-Gomez, M., and Fernandez-Decastro, A.: Plasma human placental lactogen, oxytocinase and placental phosphatase in normal and toxemic pregnancies, Am. J. Obstet. Gynecol. 127:10, 1977.
32. Hensleigh, P. A., Cheatum, S. C., and Spellacy, W. N.: Oxytocinase and human placental lactogen for prediction of intrauterine growth retardation, Am. J. Obstet. Gynecol. 129:675, 1977.
33. Rosado, A., Bernal, A., Sosa, A., Morales, M., Urrusti, J., Yoshida, F. S., Velasco, L., Yoshida, P., and Metcoff, J.: Human fetal growth retardation: III. Protein, DNA, RNA, adenine nucleotides and activities of the enzymes pyruvic and adenylate kinase in placenta, Pediatrics 50:568, 1972.
34. Urrusti, J., Yoshida, P., Velasco, L., Frenk, S., Rosado, A., Sosa, A., Morales, M., Yoshida, T., and Metcoff, J.: Human fetal growth retardation: I. Clinical features of sample with intrauterine growth retardation, Pediatrics 50:547, 1972.
35. Yoshida, T., Metcoff, J., Morales, M., Rosado, A., Sosa, A., Yoshida, P., Urrusti, J., Frenk, S., and Velasco, L.: Human fetal growth retardation: II. Energy metabolism in leukocytes, Pediatrics 50: 559, 1972.
36. Metcoff, J.: Associations between Cell Metabolism (Leukocytes) and Nutrient Status of the Mother with Fetal Malnutrition, in

Camerini-Davalos, R., and Cole, H. (eds.), *Early Diabetes in Early Life* (New York: Academic Press, 1975), p. 209.

37. Metcoff, J., Wikman-Coffelt, J., Yoshida, T., Bernal, A., Rosado, A., Yoshida, P., Urrusti, J., Frenk, S., Madrazo, R., Velasco, L., and Morales, M.: Energy metabolism and protein synthesis in human leukocytes during pregnancy and in placenta related to fetal growth, Pediatrics 51:866, 1973.

38. Crosby, W. M., Metcoff, J., Costiloe, J. P., Mameesh, M., Sandstead, H., Jacob, R. A., McClain, P. E., Jacobson, G., Reid, W., and Burns, G.: Fetal malnutrition: An appraisal of correlated factors, Am. J. Obstet. Gynecol. 128:22, 1977.

39. Merritt, T. A., Saunders, B. S., and Gluck, L.: Antenatal Assessment of Fetal Maturity: The Lung Profile, in Aladjem, S. (ed.), *Clinical Perinatology*. (In press.)

20 / Fetal Growth Retardation and Congenital Malformations

THERE SEEMS TO BE a growing consensus that a significant association exists between severe fetal growth retardation and congenital malformations.[1-8] This association has been observed among individuals not only with specific syndromes, such as Turner, Dubowitz, Russell-Silver, Down's and some of the other trisomies, but also with nonspecific types of major malformations involving musculoskeletal, cardiac, renal, cerebral and other tissues. A list of specific syndromes associated with fetal growth retardation is provided in Table 20–1. The list is based largely on information provided by Smith.[2]

The diagnosis of fetal growth retardation in individuals with either the specific types of syndromes or the nonspecific malformations generally has been made retrospectively on the basis of a very low birth weight for the infant's gestational age. There is little doubt that these individuals were undergrown in utero; they probably had short body lengths for their gestational ages. Measurements of their body lengths or head circumferences at birth rarely were available in any published reports. Their postnatal growth strongly suggests that their low birth weights were related to reductions in linear skeletal growth prenatally.

Just what is the relationship between a short stature and congenital malformations? Do all fetuses growing along the low percentiles for height have a greater risk of having congenital malformations than fetuses growing along the higher percentiles? In many ways, the published studies on nonspecific types of malformations associated with retarded fetal growth are more interesting to speculate on than the type-specific syndromes, because they seem to suggest that a general association exists between short stature and congenital malformations. Scott and Usher[3] reported an incidence of severe malformations of 17% among 60

TABLE 20–1.–SYNDROMES ASSOCIATED WITH FETAL GROWTH RETARDATION

Chromosomal abnormalities
  Aarskog
  Down
  Cri du chat
  Noonan
  Trisomy 18
  Trisomy 13
  Trisomy 8
  Turner, XO
  Williams
  XXXXY
  4p
  13q
  18p
  18q
  21q
Limb defect
  Fanconi pancytopenia
  Femoral hypoplasia—unusual facies
  Limb reduction ichthyosis
Osteochondrodysplasias
  Achondrogenesis
  Achondroplasia
  Camptomelic dwarfism
  Diastrophic dwarfism
  Ellis-van Creveld
  Grebe
  Hypochondroplasia
  Jansen metaphyseal chondrodysplasia
  Kenny
  Lymphopenic agammaglobulinemia—
    short-limbed dwarfism
  Metatropic dwarfism
  Spondyloepiphyseal dysplasia congenita
  Thanatophoric
Storage syndromes
  Generalized gangliosidosis, Type I
  Leroy I-Cell
Environmental
  Aminopterin
  Fetal alcohol
  Fetal hydantoin
  Fetal trimethadione
  Rubella
  Thalidomide
Miscellaneous
  Acrodysostosis
  Bloom
  Cerebro-costo-mandibular

TABLE 20-1.—*Continued*

Coffin-Siris
Cutis laxa—growth deficiency
DeLange
De Sanctis-Cacchione
Dubowitz
Johanson-Blizzard
Leprechaunism
Osteogenesis imperfecta
Potter
Roberts
Rothmund-Thomson
Russell-Silver
Rubinstein-Taybi
Seckel
Smith-Lemli-Opitz
Syndromes sometimes associated with
  fetal growth retardation
Cat-eye
Cytomegalic virus
Facio-auricular-vertebral
Hypophosphatasia
Meckel-Gruber
Menkes
Prader-Willi
Riley-Day
Triploidy

markedly underweight newborn infants, including congenital heart disease, myelomeningocele and hydrocephalus. Van den Berg and Yerushalmy[4] observed that 15 infants among 91 (16.5%) infants with fetal growth retardation had severe congenital malformations, including congenital heart defects, renal, gastrointestinal and cerebral malformations. Levy and co-workers[8] studied 2209 infants and children with major cardiac malformations; 6.1% of them were "small-for-dates" (low birth weight for gestational age) compared to an incidence of 2.5% in a "control" group. Studies to determine the incidence and types of congenital malformations among undergrown fetuses are complicated, because malformations often are not recognized at birth and following the postnatal courses of a given population of newborn infants in the United States is beset with dropouts. The answers to the question concerning the incidence and types of malformations among growth-retarded and normally grown fetuses are important because, as we have shown in this text, there are several well-defined maternal factors associated with severe intrauterine growth retardation that are of a remedial nature, including cigarette smoking and low weight gains by mothers during pregnancy, either as single-occurring factors or in conjunction with a short maternal height. Also, as indicated in Table 20 – 1, there are several environmental factors of a specific nature that already have been associated with the occurrence of congenital malformations in individuals with obvious fetal growth retardation. Severe fetal growth retardation is not uncommon. It is more common than indicated in published reports, because so many of the latter failed to recognize short-for-dates infants whose birth weights were above the cutoff weight arbitrarily selected. It is to be hoped that future studies will include all infants whose crown-heel lengths are abnormally short-for-dates, irrespective of their birth weights.

REFERENCES

1. Warkany, J.: *Congenital Malformations* (Chicago: Year Book Medical Publishers, Inc., 1971).
2. Smith, D. W.: *Recognizable Patterns of Human Malformation* (2d ed.; Philadelphia: W. B. Saunders Company, 1976).
3. Scott, K. E., and Usher, R.: Fetal malnutrition: Its incidence, causes and effects, Am. J. Obstet. Gynecol. 94:951, 1966.
4. Van den Berg, B. J., and Yerushalmy, J.: The relationship of the rate of intrauterine growth of infants of low birth weight to mortality, morbidity and congenital anomalies, J. Pediatr. 69:531, 1966.
5. Lugo, G., and Cassady, G.: Intrauterine growth retardation, Am. J. Obstet. Gynecol. 109:615, 1971.
6. Low, J. A., and Galbraith, R. S.: Pregnancy characteristics of intrauterine growth retardation, Obstet. Gynecol. 44:122, 1974.
7. Jones, M. D., and Battaglia, F. C.: Intrauterine growth retardation, Am. J. Obstet. Gynecol. 127:540, 1977.
8. Levy, R. J., Rosenthal, A., Tyler, D. C., and Nadas, A. S.: Birth weight of infants with congenital heart disease, Am. J. Dis. Child. 132:249, 1978.

Index

175